Chair Yoga For Seniors 10-Day Challenge

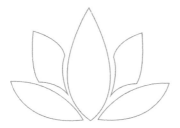

Feel 10 Years Younger in Just 10 Minutes a Day
Exercise Book + Video Workouts for Weight
Loss, Mobility, Improved Strength, and Energy

J.C. Harrison
Gran Publications

Illustrations by 🔘 Jay.Illu

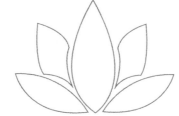

Disclaimer

This publication is provided "as is" without warranty of any kind, expressed or implied, including but not limited to warranties of performance, merchantability, fitness for a particular purpose, accuracy, omissions, completeness, currentness, or delays. The information in this book is for educational and entertainment purposes only. Efforts have been made to ensure that the content herein is accurate and up to date; however, the author and publisher make no guarantees concerning the accuracy or applicability of any content. Readers should independently verify any information within this book. The content of this book is not intended to be a substitute for professional advice. Should you require advice in a specific field, consult with a licensed professional who is qualified to provide such counsel. The author and publisher shall not be liable for any damages arising from the use, misuse, or interpretation of the information contained herein. The reader assumes full responsibility for their actions and the consequences thereof.

TABLE OF CONTENTS

INTRODUCTION

Take care of your body, it's the only place you have to live.

– Jim Rohn

Welcome to Chair Yoga for Seniors the 10-Day Challenge to Feel 10 Years Younger in Just 10 Minutes a Day. You're not just picking up a book; you're stepping into a new arena of vibrant health and independence. I'm here to guide you through this 10 day challenge that's going to help you rediscover the ease of movement in your everyday activities, like playing with your grandkids or tackling a flight of stairs, or enjoying some hobbies you used to do pain free. Over the next 10 days we are going to embrace a newfound vibrancy that transforms routine tasks into joyful experiences, all designed to enhance the quality of your life as you gracefully navigate your senior years.

Let's talk about what's in store for you by the end of this book – real, tangible benefits that go beyond the pages of this book. Imagine waking up each day with an increased sense of flexibility. Those hard-to-reach shelves? Not a problem anymore. Your body is going to feel more fluid and younger, thanks to the strength and balance you'll gain from these chair yoga poses. We're talking about real physical health benefits here – the kind that makes daily tasks a breeze and keeps you moving like clockwork.

But let's not stop there. Chronic pain and discomfort – those unwelcome guests in your life – we're going to address them head-on. If you're skeptical about how gentle movements can bring about such changes, you'll be pleasantly surprised. Through these calculated movements, you'll learn how to alleviate this pain, giving you not just relief but a renewed sense of freedom. Imagine going about your day with less pain, feeling lighter and more at ease, that's what the power of chair yoga can do for you: manage and reduce discomfort.

Your mental wellness is crucial, as a healthy body needs a healthy mind. Stress and anxiety, those mental fog creators, are going to take a back seat. This program is your ticket to a calmer, more serene state of mind. We're talking about real mood uplifts, a noticeable drop in stress levels, and an overall sense of well-being that permeates your day. Picture yourself more relaxed, more in control of your emotions, and just... happier overall.

And here's the big one that seniors tend to love getting back: independence. This program is designed to boost your ability to do things on your own, with safety and ease at its core. We're aiming to keep you independent, spry, and capable of handling your daily tasks without a hitch. Imagine the satisfaction of managing your life on your terms, with a body and mind that are fully equipped to take on the world as you enjoy your golden years.

This program isn't just about sitting in a chair and doing a few stretches. It's about igniting a transformation that touches every aspect of your life. Alongside the physical practices, you'll find educational insights about each exercise, helping you understand why and how they benefit you. This knowledge not only empowers you but also deepens the impact of each session.

As we embark on this journey together, it's important to recognize that every individual's experience with aging is unique. Whether you're a seasoned practitioner or exploring chair exercises for the first time in your senior years, this program is designed with a spectrum of abilities and health backgrounds in mind. We celebrate the diversity of our readers, understanding that each of you brings a different level of mobility, flexibility, and experience. This book aims to meet you exactly where you are, offering modifications and variations to suit your personal needs and ensure a comfortable, rewarding practice.

You're capable, you're ready, and you're about to embark on a journey that promises not just better health but a better quality of life. So, pull out your chair, take a deep breath, and get ready. Your journey to a more independent, healthy, and joyful life starts now.

HOW CHAIR YOGA SAVED MY MOM'S LIFE

Before we dive into this book and get started, I want to share the short story about my mom and how chair yoga really saved her life...

Your journey with chair exercises will be unique in its challenges and its triumphs. Some of you are looking for just an overall healthy lifestyle (easy and fun to do), others aim to reduce or eliminate arthritis pain or post-surgery pain (like my mom).

When my mom came out of her surgery, she was worried she was not going to be the same person she was before, and she was right, she wasn't. Over time and with a bit of work, she became, stronger, more agile and I am not exaggerating here, but she seemed to be younger!

Chair Yoga saved her life. She is now keeping up with her grandkids (my little ones) and going for longer walks with her friends, she was even able to start swimming again. This is what chair exercises did for my mom, and it all started with less than 10 minutes a day.

This breakthrough wasn't just a personal victory for her; it inspired her friends to make the change too. As they witnessed her transformation, their excitement to make this positive change in their lives convinced me to write what would become this book for them, and now I am sharing it with the world for the first time.

Here's a glimpse of what you can expect throughout this book:

» **Getting Ready:** Dive into the essentials first. We'll explore everything you need to start practicing chair exercises in the comfort of your home safely and enjoyably.

» **The 10 Day Challenge:** The core of our journey, featuring poses fully illustrated and selected for seniors at the beginner level. I have taken some of the best ones for beginners to start with and created the 10 Day Challenge that this book is all about.

» **The Bonus Essentials:** We go beyond the chair in the final section, venturing into nutrition and meditation. It's a straightforward and easy-to-understand guide to nourishing your body and mind, complementing the physical practices.

Why This Book Matters

This program is about more than just physical exercises; it's a comprehensive approach to improving your overall quality of life as you age. From gaining flexibility to navigating stairs with confidence and ease and of course living pain-free, it's designed to support you at all levels.

Your Expectations, My Support

What can you expect? Progress, personalized support, and someone who understands your journey. If you need one-on-one help I'm just an email away, ready to assist you at no additional charge (jcharrisonbooks@gmail.com).

Thank You for Trusting Me

Choosing this program, and me as your guide, is a privilege I hold dear. Together, let's step into this transformative expedition.

Best wishes,

J. C. Harrison

My name is JC Harrison and I couldn't be happier to work with you on this exciting new journey you are about to go on. As you have already read, this journey started with inspiration from helping my mother regain her fitness and health and more importantly helping her maintain it as she grew older.

What You've Purchased Is More Than Just a Book

You've just taken the first step with your purchase of the book, but I want you to know that you've gotten so much more! The Complete Chair Yoga Program is designed to be comprehensive and barrier-free, **offering everything you need at no extra cost.** Yes, you read that right—all the additional tools come free with your book purchase. I did this for my mother, and I'm doing it for you.

The Complete Chair Yoga Program Includes:

1. The Complete Chair Yoga Progress Tracker:

» Measuring your results is key in order to see progress, quickly and safely. I have a one-of-a-kind progress tracker that you will be able to use to track your progress throughout the length of the program.

2. HD Video Instructions :

» I have also recorded all the poses you need in easy-to-access video format. You don't need a DVD or anything, enter your email address once you have scanned the QR code or visited the website on the next page and you will get instant access. These videos will show you new ways and methods to practice chair yoga as you progress throughout the program.

3. The Chair Yoga Community For Seniors:

» Having a place where you can come ask questions and get encouragement or advice is what makes this the cornerstone of the program. We have built a fast-growing community of thousands of like-minded individuals who are looking to improve themselves and stay connected with others just like you.

4. Personalized Nutrition Plan and Meal Plan with Shopping List:

» As part of the program, you will have a fully customized nutrition and meal plan created for you. Having proper nutrition can really help speed up your results and boost your energy, so I have included that for anyone who would like to have it.

5. One on One Personalized Support:

» I am making myself available to you if you would like a slightly more personalized approach. Since I am unable to work with you in person one on one like I do with some clients, I will offer this via email for 3 months to help you hit your fitness goals. I am offering this cause I am serious about helping you reach your goals no matter what! Together anything is possible!

**TO GRAB THE REST
OF THE COMPLETE
CHAIR YOGA PROGRAM FOR FREE
SCAN HERE OR GO TO**

https://geni.us/TheChairYogaProgram

It's never too late to be what you might have been.

– George Eliot

CHAPTER 1
CHAIR YOGA
MADE SIMPLE

Finally: A Chair Program That Gets You

Let's get one thing straight: yoga isn't just about bending and stretching. It's a powerhouse for your physical and mental health. Chair yoga or as they are also often called, chair exercises (you will notice that I use both terms interchangeably in this book) takes it a notch higher for seniors, offering a cocktail of benefits tailor-made for your golden years. We're talking about increased muscle strength, skyrocketing flexibility, and balance that would make a tightrope walker jealous. But it's not just your body that gets a tune-up. Your mind gets a first-class ticket to relaxation town. Stress reduction, mental clarity, improved memory, and a mood lift are all part of the package. Imagine tackling your day with a calm mind and a body that feels like it's had a shot of youth juice. That's chair yoga for you.

Why Chair Yoga?

Think of chair yoga as yoga's more accommodating cousin. It's like yoga said, "Hey, let's make sure everyone can join in, chairs included!" Whether you're a spry 60 or a proud 90, chair yoga is your fitness pal. It adapts to your abilities, not the other way around. Got mobility issues? No problem. Chair yoga's got your back (and your knees, hips, and shoulders). It's all about making each pose work for you. The goal? To get you moving, stretching, and strengthening – all while seated. It's so adaptable, that you'll wonder why you didn't start sooner.

Seated Poses vs Standing Poses

Seated poses in chair yoga are the cornerstone of this practice, offering a blend of stability, accessibility, and focused effort. When you're seated, you've got a solid base. This means you can concentrate on each movement, each stretch, without worrying about balance. It's about engaging fully in each pose, allowing you to gently strengthen and stretch your muscles, crucial for maintaining mobility and comfort in your senior years.

Seniors over 60 benefit greatly from seated poses as they are fantastic for enhancing your core strength – yes, even while sitting! They also work wonders for your flexibility, especially in the hips and lower back, areas that can be trouble spots as we age. But it's not just about the physical. These poses are excellent for improving concentration and mental focus as well.

Think of seated poses as your foundation in chair yoga. They're where you build strength and flexibility safely, setting the stage for more challenging movements. The beauty is, they can be as gentle or as intense as you need them to be. It's yoga that truly adapts to you.

Now, let's stand up and lean into the challenge with standing poses using the chair for support. These poses are your next step in the chair yoga journey, adding an extra dimension of balance and coordination to your practice. By holding onto the chair, you're able to try poses that might otherwise be out of reach, safely expanding your range of motion and capabilities.

For people over 60 years old, the standing poses taught in this book are exceptional for enhancing lower body strength – imagine gaining firmer, more stable legs and a stronger posture this in turn will give your balance a major boost. As we age, maintaining balance becomes crucial, and these poses are your secret weapon in keeping yourself agile and confident on your feet.

Incorporating both seated and standing poses, chair yoga offers a comprehensive approach to fitness and well-being. Whether you're focusing on deep stretches while seated or challenging your balance with standing poses, you're covering the full spectrum of movement, ensuring a well-rounded, effective practice. This is chair yoga at its best – adaptable, accessible, and incredibly rewarding.

The Real Deal on Chair Yoga: Separating Fact from Fiction for Seniors

Let's cut through the noise and bust some common yoga myths, especially those that might be holding seniors back from embracing chair yoga. This isn't just about setting the record straight; it's about opening your eyes to the truth of what chair yoga can offer you.

Yoga For Any Age and Any Body

First off, the myth that yoga is only for the young and flexible? Total nonsense. Chair yoga is positive proof that yoga is for every age and every body. It's designed to be accessible and adaptable, so forget the idea that you need to be a contortionist to get started. Chair yoga meets you right where you are, whether you find yourself as stiff as a pencil or as limber as a rubber band or you haven't touched or seen your toes in decades, this practice is designed to help you gradually increase your flexibility and mobility, no matter your starting point.

And if you're thinking "I'm too old to start yoga", I'm here to tell you, there's no such thing as too old. My mother started her chair yoga journey at the ripe old age of 77. Starting chair yoga now is like planting a tree today – the best time was twenty years ago, but the second-best time is now.

Get Ready To Sweat

Now, let's tackle the misconception that chair yoga isn't a 'real workout'. If you're thinking chair yoga is just sitting around and stretching a little, think again. This is a full-body workout that can strengthen your muscles, boost your flexibility, and get your heart pumping. It's a serious exercise, with serious benefits, all from the comfort of your chair.

Low Impact, High Results

Concerned about injury or discomfort? Let's put those fears to bed. Chair yoga is low-impact and gentle on your joints, but that doesn't mean it's a walk in the park. You'll work, but you'll work safely. And remember, you're in control. If something doesn't feel right, you have the power to modify it to suit your body.

So, let's throw those old myths out the window and embrace chair yoga for what it truly is – a powerful, adaptable, and enjoyable way to boost your health, no matter your age or fitness level. It's time to take charge, get moving, and feel great doing it.

Benefits Of Chair Exercises

✓ Flexibility and Mobility

In your golden years, dealing with conditions like arthritis, osteoporosis, limited range of motion, muscle atrophy, and balance issues is common. These can make everyday movements challenging. Chair yoga comes as a savior here, offering gentle yet effective exercises to combat these ailments. Through its targeted stretches and movements, chair yoga helps ease the stiffness and pain of arthritis, improves the range of motion, counters muscle weakness, and even aids in maintaining bone health. This results in smoother, more comfortable movements in daily life, enhancing your overall mobility and flexibility.

Strength and Stability

As we age, maintaining strength and stability becomes crucial, especially when facing age-related muscle loss and balance challenges. Chair yoga is a fantastic tool for tackling these issues head-on. The practice focuses on building core strength, which is vital for overall stability and balance, reducing the risk of falls—a common concern for many seniors. Additionally, chair yoga helps in combating sarcopenia, the natural decline of muscle mass due to aging, by engaging and strengthening various muscle groups. This not only aids in daily activities like lifting and walking but also contributes to a stronger, more stable posture. By regularly practicing chair yoga, you can enhance your physical stability and strength, leading to a more confident and independent life.

Posture and Balance

For seniors, maintaining good posture and balance is vital for overall health and independence. Age-related changes can lead to a stooped posture and balance difficulties, increasing the risk of falls. Chair yoga offers a practical solution to these challenges. The poses and stretches in this chair yoga book are designed to strengthen your core and back muscles, which are essential for good posture. By reinforcing these muscles, you'll likely notice yourself standing taller and sitting straighter. Furthermore, chair yoga enhances proprioception – your body's ability to sense its position in space, which is key to maintaining balance. Regular practice can lead to significant improvements in both posture and balance, reducing the risk of falls and contributing to a sense of confidence and autonomy in your daily life.

✓ Enhanced Breathing and Circulation

Chair yoga stands as a powerful tool for seniors, especially those battling respiratory conditions like COPD and asthma. It's not just an exercise; it's your path to deeper, stronger breathing. Each breath you take becomes more powerful, combating things like high blood pressure—a frequent issue as we age.

But there's more. The movements in chair yoga are your daily boost for circulation, directly supporting your heart health. They're your answer to easing symptoms of conditions like peripheral artery disease (PAD) and chronic venous insufficiency. This is real, practical health maintenance that works. Doing chair yoga regularly can lead to better overall circulatory and respiratory health, significantly enhancing your daily comfort and activity levels.

✓ Reduced Chronic Pain

For many seniors, chronic pain is a daily reality, often due to conditions like arthritis, osteoarthritis, and fibromyalgia. Chair yoga offers a gentle yet effective way to manage and reduce this pain. Its low-impact exercises and stretches work to relieve joint stiffness and muscle tension, common culprits of chronic discomfort. The mindful movements help to increase flexibility and mobility, leading to a significant decrease in everyday aches and pains. By incorporating regular chair yoga into your routine, you can experience a noticeable reduction in chronic pain, enhancing your overall quality of life and daily functionality.

✓ Reduced Stress

Stress, a common issue among seniors, can have far-reaching effects on overall health. Chair yoga offers an effective antidote. The practice's blend of gentle physical movements and deep breathing exercises is a proven stress-buster. Engaging in these calming activities helps lower cortisol levels, the body's stress hormone, leading to a more relaxed state of mind. This stress reduction not only improves your immediate sense of well-being but also has long-term health benefits, including better heart health and improved immune function.

✓ **Improved Mental Focus and Clarity**

Chair yoga is a valuable tool in combating age-related cognitive decline, a concern for many seniors. The focused movements and breathing exercises in chair yoga engage the brain, promoting neuroplasticity – the brain's ability to form new neural connections. This engagement is crucial in maintaining and enhancing cognitive functions like memory and attention, which can diminish with age. Regular chair yoga practice can also be a proactive measure against conditions like dementia and Alzheimer's, as it keeps the brain active and engaged. Additionally, the attention and concentration required for chair yoga are beneficial for improving overall attention span, helping to mitigate age-related memory loss, and maintaining mental sharpness. By incorporating chair yoga into your routine, you can support your cognitive health, ensuring your mind remains as flexible and resilient as your body.

✓ **Boosted Mood and Overall Well-being**

Chair yoga doesn't just benefit your body and mind; it uplifts your mood too. The physical activity involved in yoga triggers the release of endorphins, the body's natural mood elevators. Additionally, the meditative aspect of yoga promotes emotional balance, helping to alleviate symptoms of depression and anxiety. Regular practitioners often report a heightened sense of overall well-being, feeling more content, optimistic, and connected to their surroundings. This positive shift in mood can transform your everyday experience, making life more enjoyable and fulfilling.

✓ Improved Quality of Sleep

As the candles on the birthday cake increase, so often do sleep disturbances. It's a common issue for those over 60, with problems ranging from insomnia to disrupted sleep patterns. Here's where chair yoga steps in as a soothing balm. The practice's relaxation and stress-reduction techniques are a direct ticket to better sleep. By calming the mind and relaxing the body, chair yoga prepares you for a deeper, more restful night's sleep. This means waking up feeling more refreshed and energized, ready to tackle the day. No more tossing and turning, just peaceful slumber.

✓ Improved Quality of Life

Growing older can sometimes mean juggling multiple health issues, from chronic pain to reduced mobility, all of which can take a toll on your quality of life. Chair yoga is like a multi-tool, designed to tackle these age-related challenges head-on. By improving flexibility, strength, balance, and mental wellness, it touches upon various aspects of your health. The result? A significant enhancement in your day-to-day living. You'll find yourself more active, more independent, and enjoying life's pleasures more fully. Chair yoga isn't just about maintaining your current state; it's about elevating your everyday experience.

✓ Can Be Done Anywhere

One of the biggest perks of chair yoga, especially for seniors, is its sheer convenience. Mobility issues or lack of access to fitness facilities can often hinder regular exercise. Chair yoga breaks down these barriers. Whether you're in your living room, at the park, or even in a small apartment, chair yoga is doable. It's adaptable to your space and needs, ensuring that maintaining your physical and mental health is always within reach, no matter where you are. This accessibility is key to building a consistent, beneficial practice that fits seamlessly into your life.

Chair Yoga for Specific Conditions and Injuries

✓ **Finding Comfort from Arthritis**

If arthritis is your constant companion, chair yoga can be a game-changer. This gentle practice targets those stiff, painful joints, bringing much-needed relief. The movements in chair yoga are designed to increase circulation and flexibility, which means less pain and more mobility in those achy joints. Imagine bending your knees to play with your grandkids or curling your fingers without that familiar twinge of pain – that's what regular chair yoga can offer. It's not just exercise; it's a form of pain relief, tailor-made for arthritis sufferers.

✓ **Stronger Bones and Osteoporosis Care**

For those battling osteoporosis, chair yoga is a beacon of hope. This low-impact exercise is gentle on the bones yet effective in maintaining bone health. The weight-bearing poses in chair yoga can help in slowing down bone density loss, a key concern with osteoporosis. What's more, the improved balance and strength from regular practice can reduce your risk of falls and fractures. It's about keeping your bones strong and your body confident, one pose at a time. In support of this, a study examining chair yoga's benefits in older adults with osteoarthritis, a condition often co-occurring with osteoporosis, found it significantly improved physical function and reduced stiffness in men and women over 60.

✓ **Soothing Strategies for Chronic Lower Back Pain Relief**

Chronic lower back pain can put a damper on your daily life as you age, but it doesn't have to. By stretching and strengthening the muscles in your lower back, chair yoga can significantly alleviate back pain. These exercises increase spinal flexibility, which means less stiffness and more ease in your everyday movements. Think about getting out of bed or standing up from a chair without that wince of pain – chair yoga can help get you there.

Supporting this, a study done demonstrated its effectiveness for older adults over 65 with chronic back pain. The research found that engaging in chair yoga improved muscular strength and flexibility, which are crucial for managing chronic back pain.

✓ Gaining Stability with Gentle Techniques for Better Balance

Balance issues can be a daunting challenge, but chair yoga stands as a reliable ally, particularly with poses like Chair Warrior II. This practice zeroes in on fortifying your core muscles and sharpening your proprioception – your innate sense of spatial awareness. The result? A notable decrease in fall risk, a primary concern for many seniors. Chair yoga isn't just about enhancing physical balance; it's about instilling confidence in each step you take, giving you the steadiness and assurance needed for everyday activities

✓ Lower Your Blood Pressure with Gentle Exercises for Hypertension Relief

High blood pressure, or hypertension, is a silent adversary, a common and serious health concern among seniors. The chair yoga exercises outlined in this book offer a powerful ally against it, providing effective strategies to manage and improve your cardiovascular health. The stress-reducing and relaxing nature of chair yoga can have a positive effect on your blood pressure levels. By engaging in deep breathing and gentle movements, you encourage your body to relax, which can naturally help lower blood pressure. It's a peaceful, pressure-reducing practice that can be a key part of your heart health strategy.

✓ Breathing Easier with COPD Using Soothing Techniques

Coping with Chronic Obstructive Pulmonary Disease (COPD) often turns simple breathing into a daily challenge. However, the routines in this program are designed to alleviate this struggle. With a strong emphasis on deep, mindful breathing, they work to improve lung capacity and respiratory efficiency, ensuring each breath you take is more effective. Diaphragmatic Breathing or Belly Breathing is one of the exercise you will learn that greatly helps with this. This method transcends traditional physical exercise, focusing on achieving ease and comfort in every breath.

✓ **Ease Anxiety and Reduce Depression with Simple Exercises**
Anxiety and depression don't have to overshadow your golden years. Here's a bright solution: the meditative and physical blend of chair yoga. This practice is a powerhouse for releasing endorphins, your body's natural mood enhancers. A study found that chair yoga helped significantly reduce anxiety and depression when practiced regularly allowing you to shift towards a more balanced emotional state. Think of it as more than just a physical workout – it's a rejuvenating boost for your mental well-being, turning each session into a step towards a happier, more balanced you.

✓ **Restoring Flexibility and Strength After Joint Replacements**
Chair yoga proves to be a crucial companion in your recovery journey after joint replacement surgery. It offers a well-structured yet gentle regimen to help you regain strength and mobility while keeping pain to a minimum. Poses like Chair Pigeon Pose specifically target the recovery of hip joints, focusing on gently stretching and opening the area to improve flexibility and reduce stiffness post-surgery.

Tailored for your healing phase, this exercise (along with many others in this book) emphasizes movements that enhance, speed up, and improve your joint flexibility and improve muscle strength, all within a safe and comfortable range. By including poses like this in your routine, you'll likely experience a decrease in discomfort and an increase in overall functionality, contributing to a faster and smoother recovery.

✓ Chair Yoga for Balancing Blood Sugar and Managing Diabetes

Let's get straight to the point: for those of you over 60 tackling type 2 diabetes, Chair Yoga is not just an exercise, it's your key best friend. Think about it – just 10 minutes of seated yoga, simple, right? Here's the deal: research shows this no-fuss routine remarkably improves your glucose control and heart health. This is about making a small change with a big impact. It's practical, doable, and incredibly effective. Incorporate Chair Yoga into your daily routine and watch it work wonders. Remember, managing diabetes isn't just about medication; it's about taking proactive steps. Chair Yoga is one such step – easy to start, hard to overlook. It's your time to show diabetes who's boss. Strong, resilient, and determined – that's you with Chair Yoga on your side.

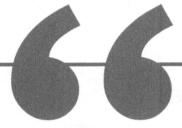

Every human being is the author of his own health or disease.

– Buddha

CHAPTER 2
SIMPLE CHAIR YOGA PREP
FOR SENIORS

Chair Yoga Made Simple

This chapter marks the beginning of a journey towards a harmonious blend of physical and mental well-being. Here, we focus on setting the stage for a transformative chair yoga experience, starting with preparing yourself mentally. It's not just about physical movement; it's about nurturing a holistic approach to health and well-being. We'll explore how to set realistic expectations, the significance of commitment, and the power of consistency in your practice.

Additionally, we will step into areas such as assessing your current physical condition, creating a safe and comfortable space for practice, and selecting the right equipment. This chapter is designed to equip you with all the necessary tools and knowledge to embark on this 10 day chair yoga challenge confidently. Get ready to embrace a practice that not only enhances your physical health but also enriches your mental and emotional well-being, one day at a time.

Mindset

Before we pull out the chair and start bending and stretching, let's set the stage mentally. Mindset preparation is key, and it's where the true transformation begins. You're not just preparing to move your body; you're gearing up to shift your entire outlook on health and well-being.

First up, setting the right **expectations**. This isn't about instant miracles or overnight transformations. It's about gradual, consistent progress. Understand that every small step you take in chair yoga is a leap toward improved health and independence. The changes you'll see and feel may start subtle – a little less stiffness here, a bit more flexibility there. But together, they add up to something profound. Expect to grow stronger and more flexible, but give it time. Patience is your friend here.

Commitment is your next cornerstone. You've got a 10 day challenge ahead of you, and it's essential to commit to this process. Think of it as a pact you're making with yourself. Each day, you'll dedicate a few minutes to your practice. It doesn't have to be lengthy; it just has to be consistent. This commitment is about showing up for yourself every day, and acknowledging that your health and well-being are worth that time. It's a powerful act of self-care and self-respect.

And that brings us to **consistency** – the real game-changer. Consistency in chair yoga isn't just about going through the motions; it's about building a habit and creating a routine that your body and mind start to crave. You'll find that the more regularly you practice, the more natural it becomes. It's like brushing your teeth – you just do it, and your day feels incomplete without it. Consistency in your practice strengthens not only your body but also your discipline and resolve. And the beauty of it? The more you do it, the more you'll want to do it. It's a positive cycle of well-being that feeds itself.

So, let's recap: Set realistic expectations – change is coming, but it's a marathon, not a sprint. Commit to the 10 day challenge – it's your commitment to better health and well-being. Be consistent – make chair yoga a non-negotiable part of your daily routine. With these mindset foundations in place, you're not just starting a fitness program; you're embarking on a journey of lifelong wellness.

With your mind primed and ready, you're all set to dive into the physical aspects of chair yoga. Let's get ready to embrace the change, one day at a time!

Understanding Your Present Physical Capabilities

Now, let's talk body. Before you dive into those poses, take a moment to assess where you're at physically. Be honest with yourself – are there aches that need nursing? Joints that need gentle coaxing? This isn't about discouraging you; it's about knowing your starting point. Understanding your current physical condition is crucial to tailor your chair yoga practice effectively. It's like setting the GPS before starting a journey; you need to know where you're starting from.

Creating a Comfortable and Safe Space

Before diving into the transformative world of chair yoga, let's focus on setting up the right environment. This section is dedicated to creating a comfortable and safe space for your practice – a fundamental step often overlooked.

Why is this important? Because your environment plays a crucial role in your chair yoga experience. It affects your concentration, comfort, and safety. This isn't just about finding a spot to place your chair; it's about creating a personal oasis where you can practice yoga without distractions or discomfort.

» **Quiet and Private Area:** Choose a spot where you won't be disturbed. This could be a corner of a room or a space where you feel relaxed and focused.

» **Enough Space:** Make sure there's enough room to move your arms and legs freely, stand up, and sit down without feeling cramped.

» **Good Lighting:** A well-lit area, preferably with natural light, is ideal. If natural light isn't available, make sure the area is brightly lit with artificial lighting.

» **Comfortable Temperature:** Ensure the room is at a comfortable temperature – not too hot or too cold.

» **Minimize Clutter:** Keep the area free from clutter to create a peaceful and safe environment.

Chair: Your Foundation for Practice

Selecting the right chair is like choosing the perfect dance partner – it needs to be just right for a harmonious experience. Your chair is the foundation of your chair yoga practice, so it's essential to choose wisely. Look for a chair that is sturdy and stable, preferably without wheels or too much cushioning, as you want to maintain a solid connection with the ground. The ideal chair doesn't have arms, allowing you the freedom to perform a wider range of movements.

The height of the chair is also crucial. When seated, your feet should rest comfortably flat on the floor, with your knees bent at a right angle. This position helps maintain proper alignment and balance as you move through various poses. A chair that's too high or too low can throw off your posture and even lead to strain or injury.

Clothing

Comfort is crucial when it comes to clothing. Wear something that allows for unrestricted movement – think stretchy, breathable fabrics. You don't need fancy yoga gear; just choose clothes that let you bend and stretch comfortably. Also, consider layers; a sweater or shawl can be handy for the relaxation portion of your practice.

Essential Props and Equipment: Utilizing Household Items

In chair yoga, you don't always need specialized equipment; many helpful props can be found right in your home. For instance, a sturdy book or a small, firm box can serve as an excellent substitute for a foam block, helping to bring the ground closer to your hands and offering support in various poses. If yoga straps aren't handy, a long belt or a scarf can work just as effectively for extending your reach and aiding in stretches. For additional comfort and support, regular household cushions or pillows can be used to prop up your hips or provide padding under your knees. A folded blanket is also versatile, perfect for extra seating support or as a cozy cover as you wrap up your session with some relaxation exercises. These everyday items are practical alternatives to traditional yoga props, making your chair yoga practice accessible, comfortable, and tailored to your needs without any extra expense.

Safety Tips

These guidelines emphasize the importance of a mindful and body-aware approach, ensuring that your chair yoga practice is both enjoyable and tailored to your individual needs and capabilities.

Breathe Fully and Slowly

Embrace deep, conscious breathing in your chair yoga practice, which is especially beneficial for seniors over 60. Proper breathing is a cornerstone of yoga, offering physical, mental, and emotional benefits that are particularly pertinent as we age. As you move through each pose with ease, reducing the likelihood of strain, you'll find that mindful breathing not only promotes physical relaxation but also enhances mental clarity and emotional well-being. This approach is gentle yet effective, catering to the changing needs of your body. It helps maintain joint flexibility, improving circulation, and boosting overall vitality. Additionally, the calming effect of deep breathing can be a valuable tool for managing age-related stress and anxiety, fostering a sense of peace and contentment that enriches your daily life

Listen to Your Body

Your body's signals are paramount. If a movement causes discomfort or pain, it's time to pull back. Yoga is about nurturing, not straining. Paying attention to your body's responses ensures a practice that is both safe and beneficial.

Keep Hydrated

Hydration is crucial, especially for seniors. Drinking water before and after your yoga session helps keep your joints lubricated and your muscles functioning optimally. It also aids in overall circulation and body temperature regulation, which as we age becomes even more important.

Stretch Gently, Avoid Overdoing

While stretching is key in yoga, overstretching can lead to injury. Approach each stretch with a sense of gentleness and caution, especially if you have existing injuries or conditions like arthritis. A mild stretch is more effective and safer than pushing too far.

✓ **Twist Slowly and Carefully**

Twists are excellent for spinal health but should be done with care. Never force a twist; your range of motion should be comfortable and pain-free. This approach helps maintain spinal integrity and prevents overstraining.

✓ **Know and Respect Your Physical Limits**

Being aware of your physical limitations is essential. If a pose feels too difficult, modify it or skip it. Chair yoga is adaptable, and there's always an alternative or modification to suit your comfort level.

✓ **Limit Time in Each Pose**

Long holds in poses can be more demanding and potentially risky, especially for beginners or those with certain health conditions. Start with shorter holds, gradually increasing as your strength and endurance improve.

✓ **Focus on Regular, Gentle Practice**

Consistency in practice is more beneficial than occasional, intense workouts. Regular, gentle chair yoga sessions are key to safely building strength and flexibility over time.

✓ **Perform Mild Backbends Only**

For those with back concerns, deep backbends might be overly intense. It's wise to opt for gentler backbends that offer a soothing stretch while being mindful not to exert excessive pressure on your spine. These milder bends help you to enjoy the benefits of flexibility and openness in your back, all while ensuring your comfort and safety. Remember, the key is to listen to your body and honor its limits, allowing for a nurturing and beneficial chair yoga practice.

✓ Avoid Pushing Yourself Too Hard

Pushing too hard in your practice can lead to fatigue and injury. Yoga is not about testing your limits but about gently expanding them. A mindful, moderate approach is always more effective and sustainable.

✓ Avoid Upside-Down Poses

Inversions (upside-down poses) are not suitable for seniors over 60, particularly for seniors who might have health concerns such as high blood pressure or glaucoma. Instead, chair yoga presents a wonderful alternative. It includes a variety of beneficial poses that can be performed safely and comfortably without the need for inversions.

My Mom's Pro Tips

As we embark on this chair yoga journey together, I want to share a few tips that really made the difference for my mom when she started Chair Yoga to help enhance your experience. These are simple but powerful ways to make the most out of your practice.

✓ Consistent Time

Finding a consistent time for your yoga practice is key. Choose a time that fits easily into your daily routine, whether it's morning or evening. Keeping a regular schedule helps in forming a habit and ensures that you're able to stick with it. It's about making yoga a regular part of your day-to-day life.

✓ Comfortable Environment

The place where you practice is important. Look for a quiet, well-lit spot in your home that's free from distractions. It doesn't have to be a large space – just somewhere you feel comfortable and can focus on your practice. Making this space inviting will help you look forward to your yoga time.

✓ Know and Understand Your Limits

It's not about pushing yourself to complete exhaustion, it's about extending your boundaries, gradually and safely. Adapting the exercises to what makes you feel safe and comfortable to help you get the best results.

✓ Free Online Coaching

To give you extra support, I'm offering free one-on-one coaching via email. If you have questions, need advice, or just want someone to check in with, I'm here for you. This coaching is a way to ensure you have all the guidance and encouragement you need to succeed in your chair yoga journey (jcharrisonbooks@gmail.com).

With these tips, I hope to help you create a fulfilling and regular chair yoga practice. It's all about finding a consistent time, setting up your space, and knowing that you have support along the way.

Before you continue!!
Make sure you download and fill out the
The Complete Chair Yoga Program Progress
Tracker. This tool will be essential for you going
forward and in helping you hit your goals.

You can find it, along with the rest of the program
for free, here:

https://geni.us/TheChairYogaProgram

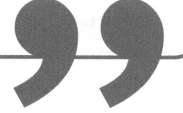

As we grow older, our bodies need more loving attention and care, not less. Movement and gentle exercise can be a beautiful expression of that care.

– Unknown

CHAPTER 3
BREATHING AND
WARM-UP EXERCISES

Diving into Chapter Three, we tackle the essentials that set the stage for a successful chair yoga practice: Breathing and Warm-Up Exercises. We will guide you through a series of beginner-friendly exercises that are crafted for seniors over 60. These aren't just preliminary steps; they are the foundation for a safe, effective, and enjoyable yoga experience. Proper breathing techniques will enhance your focus and relaxation, vital for the entire session. Warm-up exercises are equally important, as they ensure your muscles and joints are properly warmed up and ready to go minimizing the risk of injury.

As we delve into chair yoga breathing exercises, known as **Pranayama**, remember this is more than just breathing; it's an art form that enhances both your physical and mental health. These techniques are specially tailored to improve lung capacity, reduce stress, and promote relaxation, essential for the holistic health of seniors.

DIAPHRAGMATIC BREATHING

Benefits:

This technique focuses on deep breathing, a powerful practice that not only helps to alleviate stress but also contributes to lowering the heart rate and stabilizing blood pressure. By encouraging a full exchange of oxygen, it nurtures overall respiratory health. Additionally, it plays a crucial role in strengthening the diaphragm, further enhancing the efficiency of your breathing.

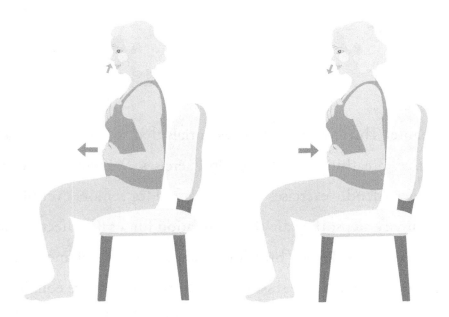

Steps:

1. Sit comfortably in a chair with your feet flat on the floor.

2. Place one hand on your chest and the other on your abdomen.

3. Inhale deeply through your nose, allowing your abdomen to rise more than your chest.

4. Exhale slowly through your mouth, feeling your abdomen fall.

5. Repeat this process for 1-3 minutes, focusing on deep, even breaths.

Benefits:

Cultivates greater lung capacity and boosts respiratory efficiency. This technique serves as a calming and grounding force, effectively clearing the mind and diminishing stress. It's also instrumental in sharpening focus and enhancing mindfulness, contributing to overall mental clarity and well-being.

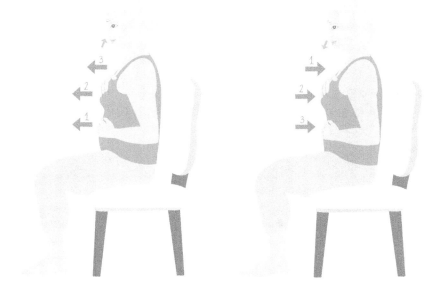

Steps:

1. Sit or lie down in a comfortable position.

2. Inhale deeply, first filling your abdomen, then your mid-chest, and finally the upper chest.

3. Exhale slowly and fully, reversing the order: empty the upper chest, mid-chest, and finally the abdomen.

4. Continue this pattern for several breath cycles, paying attention to each part of your breath.

OCEAN BREATH
(UJJAYI PRANAYAMA)

Benefits:

This breath technique is a catalyst for generating internal warmth, essential for centering and sharpening mental focus. It plays a key role in harmonizing your breath with yoga movements, creating a seamless flow. Additionally, Ujjayi Pranayama is effective in soothing the nervous system and decelerating the breath rate, fostering a sense of deep relaxation and tranquility.

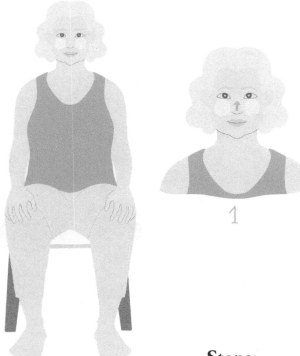

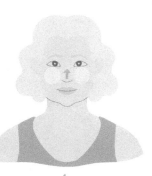

1

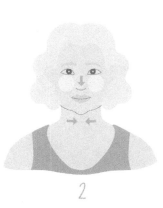

2

Steps:

1. Sit comfortably with your spine straight.

2. Inhale deeply through your nose.

3. Exhale through your nose while constricting the back of your throat, producing a soft ocean-like sound.

4. Continue this breathing, making your inhales and exhales long and steady.

Benefits:

This technique is celebrated for its ability to harmonize the left and right hemispheres of the brain. It plays a pivotal role in tranquilizing the mind, mitigating anxiety, and sharpening mental focus. Additionally, it offers significant benefits for respiratory health, enhancing overall breathing efficiency.

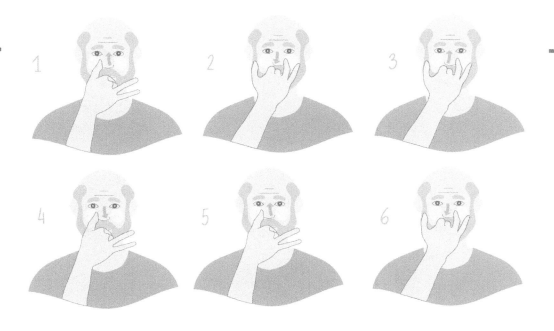

Steps:

1. Sit comfortably with a straight spine.
2. Place your left hand on your knee.
3. Use your right thumb to close your right nostril and inhale slowly through your left nostril.
4. Close your left nostril with your ring finger, release your right nostril, and exhale.
5. Inhale through the right nostril, close it, and exhale through the left.
6. Continue this alternating pattern for several minutes.

LION'S BREATH

Benefits:

Calmly soothes tension in the chest and face, and is celebrated for its revitalizing effects. It plays a significant role in easing stress and boosting circulation. Additionally, it is beneficial for throat health and enhances vocal flexibility, offering a holistic approach to well-being.

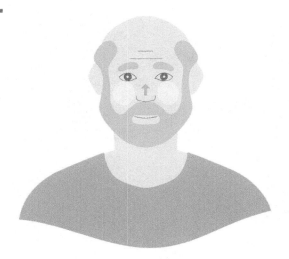
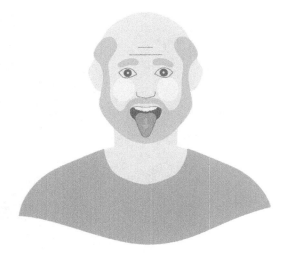

Steps:

1. Sit comfortably, inhaling deeply through your nose.
2. Exhale forcefully through your mouth, sticking out your tongue and making a 'ha' sound.
3. As you exhale, open your eyes wide and stretch the muscles of your face.
4. Repeat several times.

COOLING BREATH (SITALI PRANAYAMA)

Benefits:

As implied by its name, this technique imparts a cooling sensation throughout the body and mind. It's particularly effective in diminishing stress and soothing feelings of anger and frustration. Additionally, it plays a crucial role in regulating body temperature, making it especially valuable during hot weather or following intense physical activity.

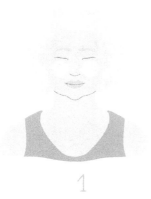
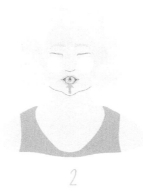
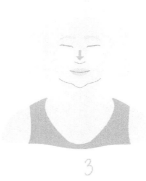

1   2   3

Steps:

1. Sit comfortably with your eyes closed.

2. Curl your tongue lengthwise and protrude it slightly past your lips.

3. Inhale through your curled tongue like sipping through a straw.

4. Close your mouth, exhaling through your nose.

5. Repeat for several breaths.

Box Breathing

Benefits:

This technique excels in stress management, as it aids in calming and stabilizing the autonomic nervous system. It also enhances concentration and sharpens focus. It's particularly valuable in high-stress scenarios or for individuals managing anxiety, providing a sense of balance and tranquility.

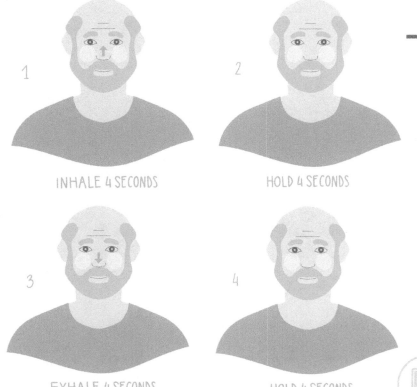

1   INHALE 4 SECONDS

2   HOLD 4 SECONDS

3   EXHALE 4 SECONDS

4   HOLD 4 SECONDS

Steps:

1. Sit upright in a relaxed position.

2. Inhale for a count of four.

3. Hold your breath for another count of four.

4. Exhale slowly for a count of four.

5. Hold your breath again for a count of four.

6. Repeat this 'box' pattern for several minutes.

Warm-up exercises and stretches help wake up the body, lubricate the joints, and ensure your chair yoga session is as safe as possible. By doing small movements you can help prepare your muscles and joints through activity similar to the poses you will be doing. This will help prevent injury and also allow you to get more from your actual chair yoga session.

Wrist & Ankle Rotation:

Rotate your wrists and ankles slowly in both directions. This helps to loosen the joints and improve circulation.

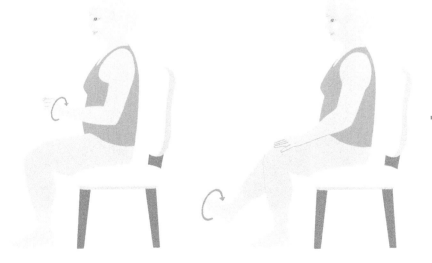

WARM-UP STRETCHES FOR BEGINNERS

Gentle Torso Twists:

Sit upright with your feet flat on the floor. Place your hands on your knees. Gently twist your torso to the right, then to the left, warming up the spine.

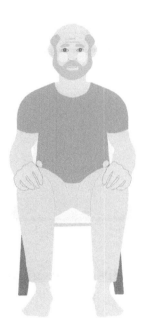
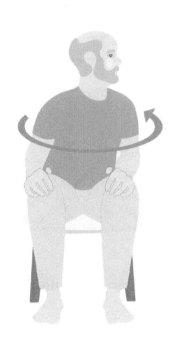
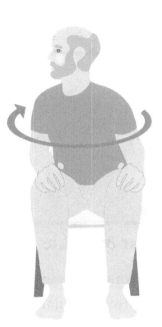

Side Neck Stretch:

Drop your right ear towards your right shoulder gently, then switch to the left side. This stretch helps to release tension in the neck muscles.

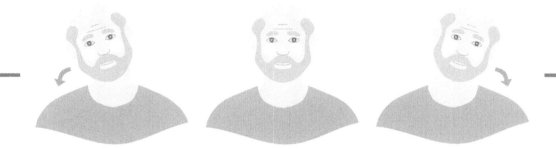

Shoulder Stretch:

Bring your right arm across your body, using your left hand to press it gently towards your chest. Switch arms after a few breaths.

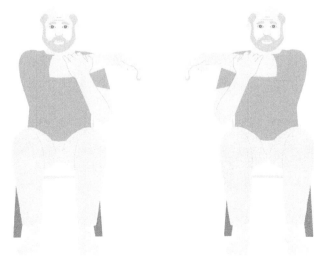

Toe and Heel Lifts:

With your feet flat on the floor, lift your toes while keeping your heels down, then lift your heels while keeping your toes down. This exercise warms up the feet and calves.

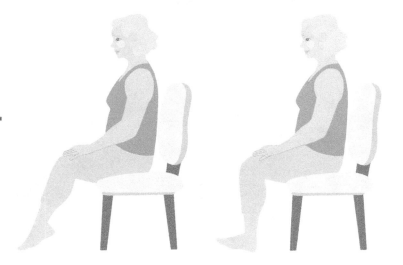

Gentle Backbend:

Place your hands on the back of your hips, gently arch your spine, and look slightly upwards, opening up the chest and front of the body.

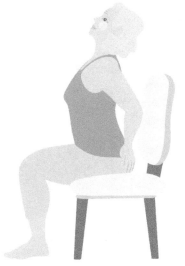

WARM-UP STRETCHES FOR BEGINNERS

Seated Neck Rolls:

Sit straight and gently lower your chin to your chest, then slowly roll your head in a circle, first to the right, then back and to the left. Repeat this motion three times, then switch directions.

1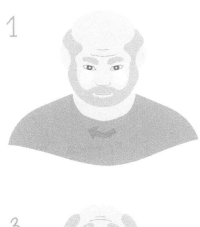

2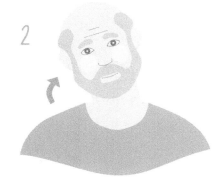

3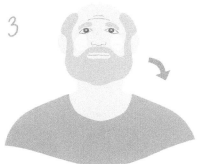

4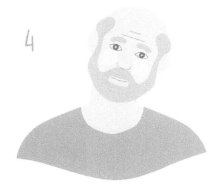

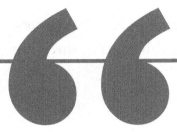

Be patient with yourself. Self-growth is tender; it's holy ground. There's no greater investment.

– Stephen Covey

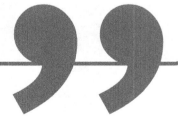

CHAPTER 4
10 DAY
CHAIR YOGA CHALLENGE

Welcome to Chapter Four, where we delve into beginner-friendly chair yoga poses specifically tailored for seniors. This chapter is all about empowering you with chair yoga poses that enhance flexibility, bolster strength, and improve balance – crucial for your golden years. You'll find each pose accompanied by clear, step-by-step instructions and illustrations as well as links to videos of the poses and tips to ensure you're practicing safely and effectively. Whether you're aiming to ease joint pain, boost circulation, or maintain mental sharpness, these poses are designed with your needs in mind.

Let me explain how the 10-day challenge will work. Each day, you'll practice a variety of poses and breathing exercises. Every few days, I'll introduce a new set of poses to keep things fresh while giving you time to improve on the individual poses.

- **Days 1 - 3**: Build Your Foundation. In the first week, we'll kick things off with the essential poses. You'll focus on mastering these moves, building a solid foundation, and getting comfortable with the basics. No rush, just steady progress.

- **Days 4 - 6**: Keep It Fresh. As we move into the week, we switch up the poses. This keeps things exciting and ensures you don't get bored. Variety is key to keeping your body engaged and your mind motivated.

- **Days 7 - 8**: Challenge and Progressing. is all about pushing a bit further. We'll introduce new poses that build on what you've already learned, increasing the challenge just enough to keep you progressing.

- **Days 9 - 10**: Mastery and Results. By the final days, you'll be incorporating a variety of poses into your routine. You'll notice a significant decrease in pain and a newfound confidence in your abilities. You're not just getting comfortable with chair yoga – you're mastering it.

Stick with it, stay consistent, and by the end of these first 10 days, most people say they feel 10 years younger! If you don't, don't worry it just means your body is taking a bit long to adjust. Take a one day break and redo the exercises starting from day one and make sure you join our Facebook group to let us know that you completed your 10 day challenge. Let me show you all the poses that we will cover and then at the end of this chapter, I will lay out the plan for you to follow!

GENTLE NECK ROLL AND STRETCH

Benefits:

This gentle exercise is designed for seniors to relieve neck tension and improve flexibility. By focusing on the neck muscles, it offers a soothing stretch that can enhance mobility and comfort in the neck area.

Safety Precautions:

• Perform movements gently to avoid strain.

• If you experience dizziness, pause and return to a neutral position.

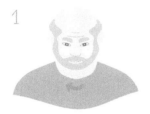 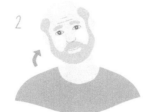 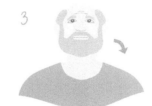 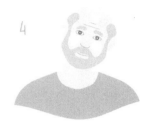

Steps:

1. Begin by sitting in a comfortable chair with your spine aligned and upright. This posture ensures a safe foundation for the exercise.

2. Slowly tilt your head forward, guiding your chin towards your chest. This initial movement starts the stretch and begins to release tension in the neck.

3. Gently roll your head to the right, aiming to bring your ear closer to your shoulder. This action stretches the side neck muscles, aiding in flexibility.

4. Continue the motion by rolling your head backward and then to the left, completing a smooth, circular movement. This sequence helps to evenly distribute the stretch across the neck muscles.

5. Perform 3-5 rolls in each direction, moving at a pace that feels comfortable and safe. Ensure each roll is performed gently to avoid any strain.

SHOULDER SHRUGS

Benefits:

Excellent for relieving tension in the shoulders and neck, while improving upper body mobility. This simple yet powerful movement targets the shoulders and upper back, promoting relaxation and flexibility in these areas.

Safety Precautions:

- Move slowly and avoid overexerting the shoulder muscles.

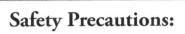

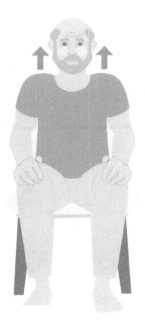

Steps:

1. Sit upright in a chair with your feet firmly planted on the floor. This stable base supports proper posture and alignment throughout the exercise.

2. Inhale deeply, and with intention, lift your shoulders towards your ears. This upward movement should be controlled, engaging the muscles without straining them.

3. As you exhale, consciously release your shoulders back down. This downward motion encourages relaxation and the release of any built-up tension.

4. Repeat the shrugging motion 5-10 times, focusing on smooth, deliberate movements. Each shrug should contribute to a greater sense of ease in your shoulders and neck.

Targeted Areas:
Spine and abdominal muscles.

CHAIR ASSISTED TORSO TWISTS

Benefits:

An effective way to enhance spinal mobility, alleviate back stiffness, and support digestive health.

Safety Precautions:

• Twist gently, avoiding any forceful movements.

• If you have a spine condition, consult a healthcare professional first.

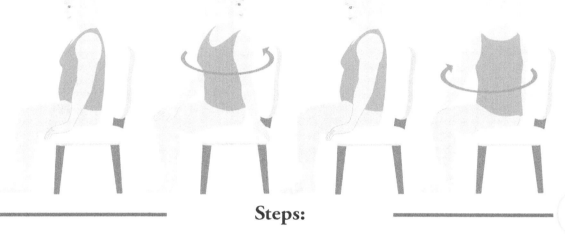

Steps:

1. Begin by sitting upright in a chair, ensuring your feet are flat on the ground. This position helps maintain balance and proper spinal alignment during the twist.

2. Place your right hand on your left knee and your left hand behind you on the chair. These hand placements provide stability and support for the twist.

3. Inhale deeply to prepare. As you exhale, gently twist your torso to the left. This movement should originate from the base of your spine, ensuring a gentle and effective stretch.

4. Hold the twist for a few breaths, allowing your body to relax into the position. This holding phase aids in deepening the stretch while supporting spinal health and digestion.

5. Slowly return to the center before repeating the exercise on the opposite side. This ensures balanced mobility and flexibility on both sides of the body.

SEATED SPINAL EXTENSION

Targeted Areas:
Lower and upper back.

Benefits:

Strengthens back muscles, enhancing posture, and increasing spinal flexibility.

Safety Precautions:

• Do not overextend your back.
• Move into the position slowly and smoothly.

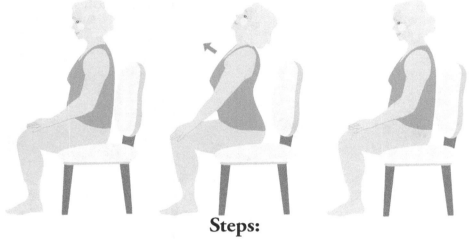

Steps:

1. Sit at the edge of a stable chair with your feet firmly planted on the ground. This starting position ensures a solid foundation for the exercise.

2. Place your hands on your thighs for support. This helps maintain balance and alignment as you move through the spinal extension.

3. Inhale deeply and gently begin to arch your back. Push your chest forward and draw your shoulders back, engaging the muscles along your spine.

4. Hold this arched position for a few seconds, allowing your back muscles to stretch and strengthen. Be mindful not to overextend; the movement should be comfortable and controlled.

5. Exhale slowly and return to your starting position, feeling the length and relaxation in your spine.

6. Repeat the exercise 5-7 times, focusing on smooth, deliberate movements. Each repetition will contribute to a greater sense of strength and flexibility in your back.

Targeted Areas:
Lateral muscles, obliques, and ribcage.

SEATED SIDE STRETCH

Benefits:

Improves flexibility and can help reduce stiffness in the sides and back, contributing to overall comfort and mobility.

Safety Precautions:

• Stretch only as far as comfortable.

• Avoid this exercise if you have severe rib or spine issues.

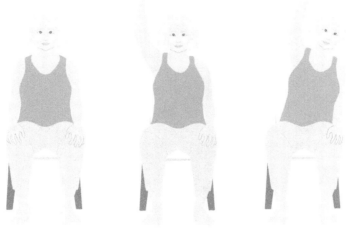

Steps:

1. Start by sitting upright in a chair with your feet flat on the ground, establishing a stable and comfortable base.

2. Inhale and raise your right arm overhead, ensuring your posture remains straight and aligned.

3. As you exhale, gently lean to the left. This movement stretches the right side of your body, from the ribcage to the obliques. Move into the stretch only as far as feels comfortable, avoiding any strain.

4. Hold the position for a few breaths, allowing the stretch to deepen with each exhale. This not only enhances the stretch but also aids in relaxation.

5. Slowly return to the center and lower your arm. Then, repeat the stretch on the left side, raising your left arm and leaning to the right.

SEATED WARRIOR II ARMS

Targeted Areas:
Arms, shoulders, and upper back.

Benefits:

A fantastic way to fortify and stretch arms and shoulders while also sharpening your focus.

Safety Precautions:

• Keep the shoulder blades down and back to avoid tension.

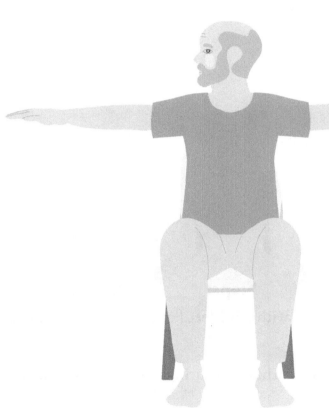

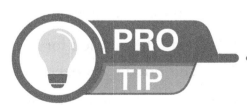

SEATED WARRIOR II ARMS

Steps:

1. Begin by sitting upright in a chair, ensuring your feet are flat on the ground. This stable base aids in maintaining proper posture throughout the exercise.

2. Stretch your arms out to either side, reaching them to shoulder height with your palms facing down. This action engages the muscles in your arms and shoulders, promoting strength and flexibility.

3. Turn your head to gaze over your right hand, extending the stretch and enhancing your focus. This not only helps in stretching the neck muscles but also aids in concentration and mental clarity.

4. Hold this position for several deep breaths, encouraging a deeper engagement with each exhale. Ensure your shoulder blades are drawn down and back to prevent any unnecessary tension in your neck and shoulders.

5. Gently bring your gaze back to the center before turning to look over your left hand, effectively repeating the pose on this side. This ensures a balanced stretch and strength enhancement across both sides of your body.

"Explore Micro-Movements"

In each pose, experiment with subtle shifts—tilting your pelvis, adjusting your shoulder blades, or turning your palms. These micro-movements can deepen the pose's effect and increase body awareness.

Targeted Areas:
Arms and shoulders.

SEATED ARM CIRCLES

Benefits:

Improve shoulder mobility, increase upper body strength, and enhance circulation.

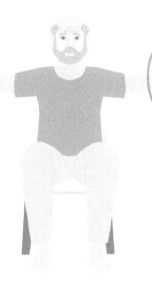

Safety Precautions:

• Keep your movements slow and controlled to avoid any strain on your shoulders.

• If you experience any pain or discomfort, reduce the size of your circles or take a break.

Steps:

1. Begin by sitting upright in a chair, with your feet flat on the ground.

2. Extend your arms out to the sides at shoulder height, keeping them straight. Ensure your palms are facing down to start, positioning your body in a T-shape.

3. Start making small circles with your arms, moving them in a forward motion. Focus on keeping the circles controlled and your arms level with your shoulders.

4. Gradually increase the size of the circles as you become more comfortable, ensuring you maintain control and do not strain your shoulder muscles.

5. After 15 seconds or when you're ready, reverse the direction of your circles, moving your arms in a backward motion. This change helps to engage different muscles.

6. Continue performing the arm circles for a total of 30 seconds to 1 minute, alternating between forward and backward motions.

CHAIR CAT-COW STRETCH

Targeted Areas:
Spine, neck, and shoulders.

Benefits:

This gentle movement helps increase spine flexibility and relieve tension in the back and neck. It can also aid in improving posture and breathing.

Safety Precautions:

• Move slowly and gently to avoid any strain.

• If you have severe back pain or a spinal injury, consult with a healthcare provider before attempting this exercise.

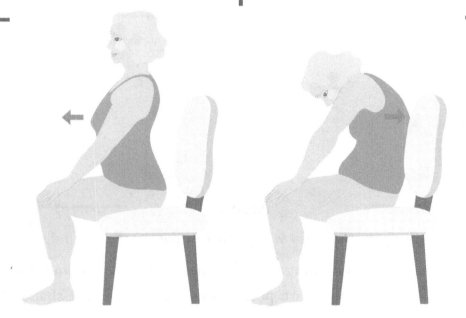

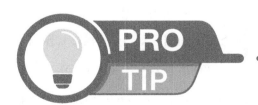

Steps:

1. Sit upright towards the front edge of a stable chair, placing your feet flat on the floor, hip-width apart. Place your hands on your knees or thighs for support.

2. Begin with the Cow pose: Inhale, arch your back, and tilt your pelvis back, sticking your buttocks out slightly. Lift your chest and chin upwards, gazing slightly forward or up, and pull your shoulders back. This position encourages a gentle arch in your lower back, opening the chest and stretching the front of your torso.

3. Transition to the Cat pose: Exhale, round your spine, and tilt your pelvis forward, tucking your tailbone under. Draw your chin towards your chest, gaze down at your navel, and push your mid-back towards the chair back. This movement stretches the back of your spine and releases tension in your neck and shoulders.

4. Continue to flow smoothly between the Cow and Cat poses, following the rhythm of your breath: Inhale as you move into Cow pose, and exhale as you transition into Cat pose.

5. Repeat this sequence for several breath cycles (typically 5-10), focusing on the sensation of movement along your spine and the relaxation of tension with each transition.

"Engage Your Senses"

Integrate aromatherapy or calming sounds into your practice environment. A drop of lavender oil on your wrists or calming nature sounds can deepen relaxation and enhance the sensory experience of your practice.

SEATED SHOULDER ROLLS

Targeted Areas:
Shoulders, neck, and upper back

Benefits:

This simple yet effective exercise is designed to release tension in the shoulders and neck, improve mobility, and enhance posture.

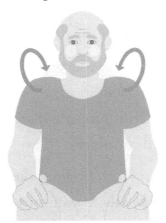

Safety Precautions:

- Perform the movements slowly and gently to avoid any strain.
- Keep your spine straight and aligned to prevent slouching during the exercise.
- Breathe naturally, coordinating your breath with the movement for maximum relaxation.

Steps:

1. Begin sitting upright in a chair with your feet flat on the floor, hip-width apart. Place your hands on your thighs or let them hang by your sides.

2. Inhale deeply, and as you exhale, slowly lift your shoulders towards your ears.

3. Continue the movement by gently rolling your shoulders back, drawing your shoulder blades towards each other to open up the chest.

4. As you complete the backward roll, lower your shoulders, creating a circular motion.

5. Once your shoulders are in their lowest position, begin the next roll by lifting them towards your ears again, then forward, up, back, and down, reversing the direction.

6. Perform this circular motion slowly and smoothly for several repetitions, typically 5-10 times in each direction, focusing on the sensation of release and relaxation in your shoulder and neck area.

7. Pause for a moment after completing the rolls in both directions, taking a few deep breaths to settle into the relaxation and openness created by the exercise.

Targeted Areas:
Torso, hips and lower back.

SEATED TORSO CIRCLES

Benefits:

A gentle yet effective exercise for seniors, aimed at increasing hip and lower back mobility and alleviating stiffness in these areas.

Safety Precautions:

• Ensure the chair is stable.

• Avoid this exercise if you have severe hip pain.

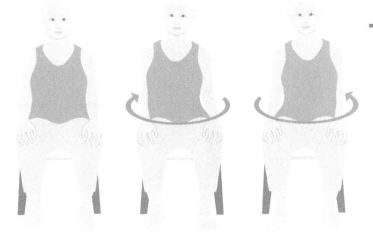

Steps:

1. Begin by sitting near the edge of a stable chair. Place your feet firmly on the floor, hip-width apart, establishing a strong foundation.

2. Rest your hands on your hips for added stability. This also helps in maintaining an upright posture throughout the exercise.

3. Initiate the movement by gently guiding your upper body in a circular motion to the right. Ensure the motion originates from the torso, engaging the muscles around the hip joint and lower back.

4. Continue the circular motion, moving your torso back, then to the left, and finally bringing them forward. This motion should be fluid and controlled, focusing on the range of motion that feels comfortable.

5. Complete five circles in this direction, then reverse the direction for another five circles. The reversal ensures balanced mobility & muscle engagement on both sides.

CHAIR ASSISTED LEG LIFTS

Targeted Areas:
Thighs and core.

Benefits:

Strengthen the thighs while also enhancing stability and balance.

Safety Precautions:

- Move slowly and control the movement.
- Do not overextend if you have knee problems.

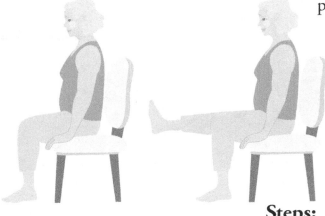

Steps:

1. Begin by sitting upright in a stable chair, ensuring your feet are flat on the ground. This starting position promotes good posture and prepares your body for the exercise.

2. Grasp the sides of the chair lightly for support. This not only aids in maintaining balance during the exercise but also ensures safety and control.

3. Carefully extend one leg out in front of you, striving to keep it parallel to the floor. The goal is to activate the muscles in your thigh and core without straining them.

4. Hold this extended position for a few seconds, focusing on engaging the thigh muscles while keeping the rest of your body stable.

5. Gently lower the leg back to the starting position, controlling the movement to maximize the exercise's benefits.

6. Perform 5-10 repetitions with each leg, alternating to ensure balanced strength and flexibility in both legs.

Benefits:

An excellent exercise for focusing on stretching the spine and lower back. It not only eases tension in these areas but also aids in calming the mind.

Safety Precautions:

- Bend from your hips, not your waist.
- Avoid if you have severe lower back issues.

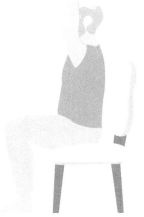
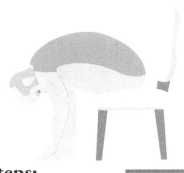

Steps:

1. Start by sitting upright on a secure chair. Keep your feet planted on the floor, ensuring they are parallel and hip-width apart for stability.

2. Inhale deeply and raise your arms overhead, bringing a gentle stretch to your upper body. This upward movement also aids in elongating the spine.

3. As you exhale, gradually hinge forward from your hips, not the waist. This distinction is crucial for targeting the right muscles and ensuring safety.

4. Extend your hands towards your feet or shins, depending on your comfort and flexibility. The key is to stretch without straining.

5. Hold for a few deep breaths, allowing the stretch to penetrate your spine and lower back. Focus on the sensation of release in your back with each exhale.

6. Slowly rise back to the sitting position, using your hands for support if necessary.

SEATED CALF RAISES

Benefits:

Aimed at strengthening the calf muscles and improving ankle stability. This exercise is crucial for maintaining mobility, balance, and support during daily activities.

Safety Precautions:

• Move slowly and avoid jerky movements.

• If you have ankle or calf injuries, proceed with caution.

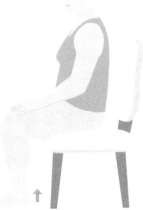
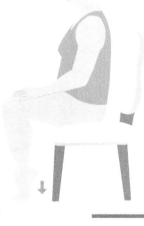

Steps:

1. Start by sitting upright in a chair with your feet flat on the floor. Ensure your posture is straight, supporting overall alignment and balance.

2. Gradually raise your heels off the floor, shifting your weight onto the balls of your feet. This movement engages the calf muscles, promoting strength and stability.

3. Hold this raised position for a few seconds. This pause is key to maximizing muscle engagement and enhancing stability in the ankles.

4. Gently lower your heels back to the floor, controlling the movement to ensure smooth and steady strengthening.

5. Repeat the calf raise 10-15 times. This repetition range is optimal for building strength and endurance in the calf muscles and ankles.

CHAIR TREE

Targeted Areas:
Legs, ankles, and core.

Benefits:

A chair yoga pose that focuses on improving balance, strengthening the ankles and calves, and enhancing focus.

Safety Precautions:

• Avoid if you have severe knee or hip problems.

OPTIONAL

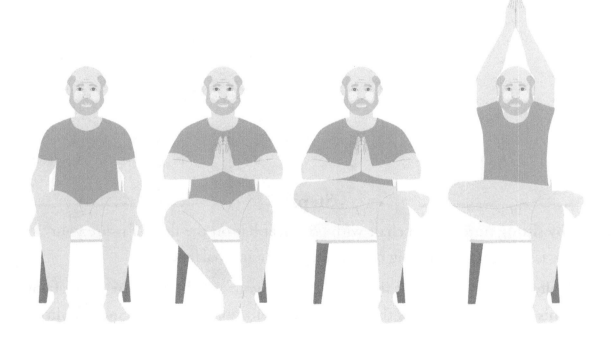

Steps:

1. Begin by sitting upright in a stable chair, with your feet firmly planted on the floor. This position ensures proper posture and balance from the start.

2. Carefully place your right foot on top of the left thigh, making sure to avoid resting it directly on the knee joint. For a less intense variation, rest your right foot on your left ankle instead.

3. Gently press your right knee towards the floor to open up the hip. This movement should be done gently to avoid strain, focusing on the stretch and opening of the hip.

4. Bring your hands together in a prayer position at your chest or, for an added challenge, raise them overhead, keeping your shoulders away from your ears. This adds an element of balance and focus to the pose.

5. Hold this position for 5-10 breaths, focusing on maintaining balance and stability. The breath will aid in concentration and steadiness.

6. After completing one side, gently release and switch sides, repeating the process with the left foot on the right thigh or ankle.

SEATED LEG STRETCHES

Targeted Areas:
Hamstrings, calves, and lower back.

Benefits:

It enhances flexibility in the hamstrings and lower back, crucial for improving mobility and easing daily movements.

Safety Precautions:

- Do not overstretch; go only as far as comfortable.

- Avoid if you have severe sciatica.

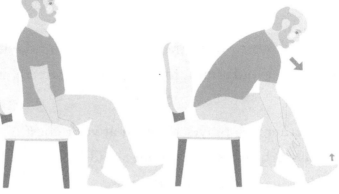

Steps:

1. Start by sitting on the edge of a stable chair, ensuring your posture is upright. This initial position helps maintain balance and alignment for an effective stretch.

2. Fully extend one leg forward, resting the heel on the ground and toes pointing upwards. If you find it challenging, it's perfectly fine to keep a slight bend in the knee. This position targets the hamstring and calf of the extended leg.

3. Keep the other foot flat on the floor to support balance and stability.

4. Inhale deeply to prepare. As you exhale, gently lean forward from your hips towards the extended leg. This forward motion enhances the stretch in the hamstring and lower back. Move into the stretch only as far as comfortable, avoiding any strain.

5. Hold the position for a few breaths, allowing the stretch to deepen gently with each exhale. This not only aids in flexibility but also promotes relaxation.

6. After holding, gently return to the starting position and switch legs, repeating the stretch to ensure balanced flexibility on both sides.

Targeted Areas:
Spine, abdominal muscles, and back.

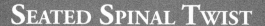

Benefits:

An effective exercise designed to enhance spinal mobility, relieve back stiffness, and support digestion and stress relief.

Safety Precautions:

• Twist gently, avoiding any forceful movements.

• If you have a spine condition, consult a healthcare professional first.

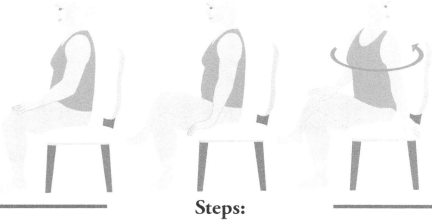

Steps:

1. Begin by sitting upright on a stable chair, with your feet flat on the floor.

2. Cross your left leg over your right, placing your left foot beside your right knee. This setup prepares your body for a deeper twist and stretch.

3. Place your right hand on your left knee and your left hand behind you on the chair. These hand placements aid in supporting the twist and ensuring stability.

4. Inhale deeply to prepare your body. As you exhale, gently twist your torso to the left, aiming to look over your left shoulder. This movement initiates the twist from your lower back, extending up through your spine to your neck.

5. Hold the position for a few breaths, allowing the twist to deepen gently with each exhale. Focus on feeling the stretch throughout your spine.

6. After holding, slowly return to the center before repeating the exercise on the opposite side. This ensures balanced flexibility and mobility in both directions.

SEATED KNEE LIFTS

Targeted Areas:
Thighs and hips.

Benefits:

Focuses on strengthening thigh muscles and improving hip mobility.

Safety Precautions:

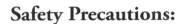

- Lift the knee only as high as comfortable.
- Avoid if you have acute hip pain.

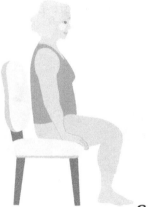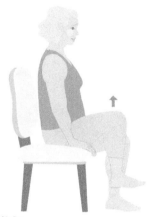

Steps:

1. Begin by sitting upright on a stable chair, ensuring your feet are flat on the ground. This starting posture helps maintain balance and alignment during the exercise.

2. Place your hands on your thighs or the sides of the chair for additional stability. This support is crucial for maintaining proper form throughout the movement.

3. Slowly lift one knee towards your chest, keeping the movement controlled and the other foot flat on the floor. This action engages the thigh muscles and encourages hip mobility.

4. Hold the lifted position for a few seconds, focusing on engaging your core and thigh muscles. This hold increases muscle strength and stability.

5. Gently lower the leg back to the starting position, ensuring the movement is smooth and controlled.

6. Alternate legs, performing 10-15 lifts per leg. This repetition ensures balanced strength and flexibility in both hips and thighs.

Targeted Areas:
Calves and feet.

Benefits:

Excellent exercise for those looking to enhance lower leg strength, boost circulation, and improve coordination.

Safety Precautions:

• Tap gently to avoid jarring your legs.

• Suitable for those with limited lower body mobility.

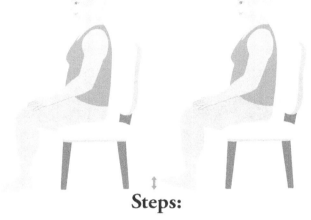

Steps:

1. Position yourself upright in a chair, ensuring your feet are placed flat on the ground. This posture ensures stability and alignment as you perform the toe taps.

2. Engage your leg muscles to lift your toes while keeping your heels firmly planted on the floor. This action begins the strengthening and circulation enhancement in the lower legs.

3. Gently tap your toes back down to the floor, creating a rhythmic motion. The tapping not only strengthens the muscles but also promotes coordination and agility in the feet and calves.

4. Continue this tapping motion for 20-30 seconds, maintaining a steady pace. Focus on the movement of lifting and lowering the toes, ensuring each tap is controlled and deliberate.

5. Throughout the exercise, keep your posture upright and your movements smooth to maximize the benefits and minimize any risk of strain.

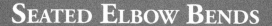

Targeted Areas:
Arms, especially biceps and triceps.

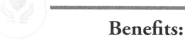

Benefits:

This exercise strengthens the arms and improves elbow joint mobility.

Safety Precautions:

• Move in a controlled manner.

• If you have elbow or shoulder pain, proceed cautiously.

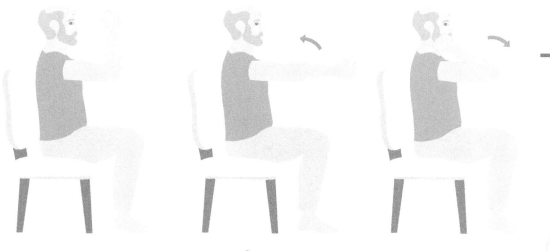

Steps:

1. Sit upright on a chair, ensuring stability and proper posture. This initial position is key for alignment and effectiveness of the exercise.

2. With arms extended forward and elbows bent at a 90-degree angle, you're positioned to begin the strengthening movement.

3. Smoothly extend your arms straight, then bend the elbows to bring your fists towards your shoulders. This motion engages the arm muscles in a controlled manner.

4. Repeat this bending and extending action 10-15 times, focusing on a fluid movement to maximize muscle engagement and joint mobility.

5. The controlled pace helps in focusing on muscle strength and joint flexibility, making each repetition effective.

CHAIR SUN SALUTATION

Targeted Areas:
Full body, including spine, arms, and legs.

Benefits:

A comprehensive exercise that enhances overall flexibility, boosts energy, and improves breathing.

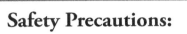

Safety Precautions:

• Move through each step smoothly and avoid overstretching.

• Be mindful of your breathing.

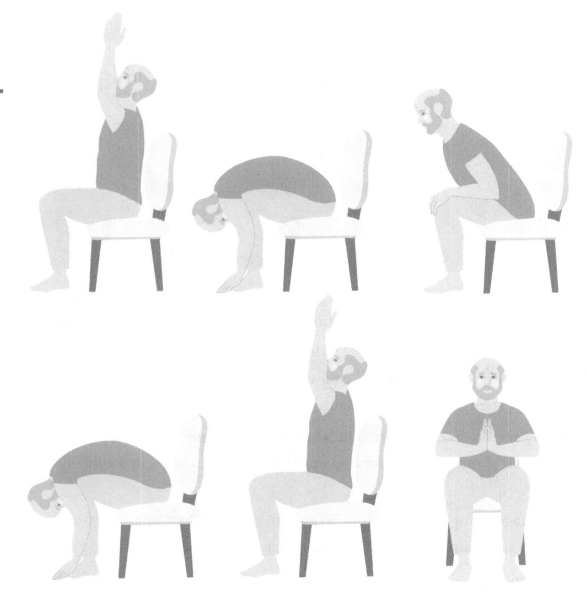

CHAIR SUN SALUTATION

Steps:

1. Position yourself upright in a chair with your feet firmly planted on the ground, establishing a stable foundation.

2. Inhale deeply and raise your arms overhead, directing your gaze upwards, inviting energy and openness into your body.

3. Exhale and fold forward from the hips, extending your hands towards your feet. This forward bend encourages flexibility in the spine and legs.

4. Inhale and lift your torso halfway up, achieving a straight back. This movement helps to lengthen the spine and refresh the posture.

5. Exhale and fold forward again, deepening the stretch and promoting relaxation.

6. With another inhalation, rise up smoothly, stretching your arms overhead once more, embracing a full body stretch.

7. Exhale and bring your hands to your heart, centering your energy and focus as you conclude the sequence.

8. Repeat this sequence 3-5 times, flowing through each step with mindfulness and ease.

SEATED KNEE EXTENSIONS

Targeted Areas:
Thighs and knees.

Benefits:

Excellent way to strengthen thigh muscles and enhance knee joint mobility.

Safety Precautions:

- Extend your knee gently.
- Avoid if you have severe knee pain.

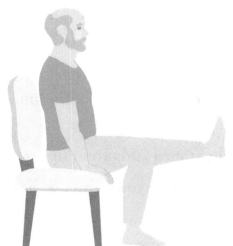

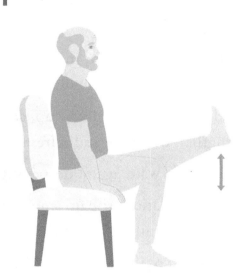

Steps:

1. Begin by sitting upright on a chair, ensuring your feet are firmly on the ground.

2. Extend one leg out in front of you, preparing for the lift. This action sets the stage for strengthening the muscles around your knee.

3. Slowly raise and lower the extended leg, maintaining a smooth and controlled movement. This precision helps in maximizing muscle engagement while protecting the knee joint.

4. Aim for 10-15 lifts, focusing on the quality of movement rather than speed. Each lift contributes to building strength in the thigh muscles and improving flexibility in the knee joint.

5. After completing the set, switch to the other leg to ensure balanced strengthening across both legs.

Targeted Areas:
Thighs, hips, and buttocks.

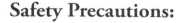
CHAIR ASSISTED SQUATS

Benefits:

Excellent exercise for those looking to enhance lower leg strength, boost circulation, and improve coordination.

Safety Precautions:

• Squat only as low as comfortable.

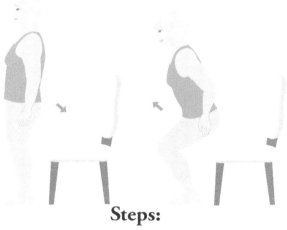

Steps:

1. Begin by standing in front of a stable chair, ensuring it's securely positioned to support you if needed. Your feet should be hip-width apart, aligning your body for optimal movement.

2. Initiate the squat by slowly lowering your body, as if intending to sit down. This movement engages the muscles in your thighs, hips, and buttocks, building strength and flexibility.

3. Bend at the knees and hips, keeping your chest upright and core engaged. This posture ensures a safe, effective squat that targets the right areas without strain.

4. Before making contact with the chair, press through your heels to stand back up. This phase of the exercise challenges your balance and strength, enhancing stability.

5. Aim to complete 10-15 repetitions, maintaining a smooth, controlled motion throughout. Each squat should be performed with care, focusing on form and comfort.

SEATED JUMPING JACKS

Targeted Areas:
Full body, especially the arms and legs.

Benefits:

A low-impact alternative to traditional jumping jacks, perfect for seniors seeking to increase their heart rate, improve cardiovascular health, and boost coordination.

Safety Precautions:

- Move in a controlled manner.
- If you have joint issues, be cautious with the movements.

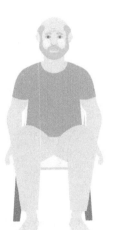

Steps:

1. Begin by sitting upright in a chair, legs together, and arms resting at your sides. Activate your lower abdominal muscles to reduce strain on your back. This starting position ensures stability and readiness for the movement.

2. With a smooth, coordinated motion, extend your legs simultaneously raising your arms above your head. This action mimics the dynamic motion of standing jumping jacks, engaging multiple muscle groups.

3. Carefully return to the starting position, maintaining control and balance throughout the movement. This return phase is crucial for coordinating the exercise and ensuring safety.

4. Aim for 10-20 repetitions, adjusting the number based on your comfort and fitness level. Each repetition should be performed with intention, focusing on controlled movements to maximize benefits while minimizing the risk of strain.

Targeted Areas:
Core, lower abdominals, and hip flexors.

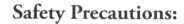

CHAIR FLUTTER KICKS

Benefits:

Focuses on strengthening the core and lower abdominal muscles while also improving leg mobility.

Safety Precautions:

• Move in a controlled manner to prevent lower back strain.

• Suitable for those with a moderate level of abdominal strength.

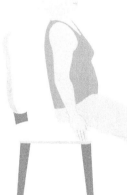

Steps:

1. Begin by sitting on the edge of a chair. This position allows you to maintain balance and ensures the effectiveness of the exercise. Lean slightly back, but ensure your spine remains aligned to avoid any strain on your back.

2. Hold onto the sides of the chair for support. This grip will help you maintain your balance and position as you perform the flutter kicks.

3. Extend your legs in front of you, raising them slightly off the floor. Keep your legs straight, engaging your core muscles to support the movement.

4. Start to alternately lift each leg in a small, fluttering motion. This action should be controlled and steady, focusing on engaging the lower abdominals and hip flexors with each flutter.

5. Continue the flutter kicks for 30 seconds to 1 minute, depending on your comfort and ability. The goal is to maintain a steady pace and controlled movement throughout the exercise to maximize the benefits while minimizing the risk of strain.

Targeted Areas:

Chest, shoulders, and upper back.

SEATED CHEST OPENER

Benefits:

Designed to improve posture, open up the chest, and alleviate respiratory discomfort. This exercise promotes a more upright posture and facilitates easier breathing.

Safety Precautions:

• Avoid overextending your back.

• If you have lower back issues, proceed cautiously.

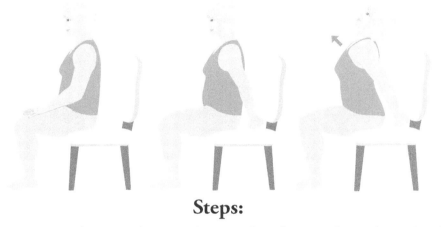

Steps:

1. Begin by sitting upright in a chair with your feet firmly planted on the floor. This stable position ensures proper alignment and support throughout the exercise.

2. Clasp your hands behind your back. This action prepares your upper body for the stretch and helps in engaging the correct muscles.

3. Inhale deeply, and as you exhale, gently pull your clasped hands downwards. Simultaneously, open your chest and lift your gaze slightly upwards. This movement stretches the chest and shoulders, encouraging a natural opening of the upper body.

4. Hold this position for several breaths, allowing the stretch to deepen with each exhale. The focus should be on maintaining a gentle stretch that opens the chest without straining the back.

5. Carefully release the stretch and relax. The controlled return to a relaxed state helps in maximizing the benefits of the stretch while ensuring safety.

SEATED EAGLE ARMS

Targeted Areas:
Shoulders, upper back, and arms.

Benefits:

Designed to increase shoulder mobility, stretch the upper back, and relieve tension in the neck and shoulders.

Safety Precautions:

- Do not strain your shoulders; keep the movement gentle.
- Avoid if you have severe shoulder pain.

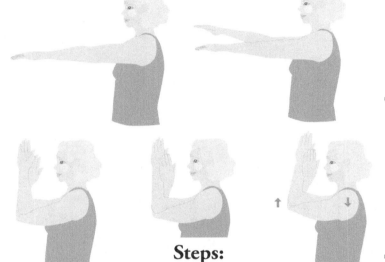

Steps:

1. Begin by sitting upright, ensuring your feet are firmly planted on the ground. This position stabilizes your base, allowing for a focused stretch in the upper body.

2. Extend your arms straight in front of you at shoulder height, preparing your muscles.

3. Cross your right arm over your left, bend your elbows and twist your forearms until your palms meet. This alignment targets the stretch in the shoulders and upper back.

4. Gently lift your elbows while consciously lowering your shoulders away from your ears. This deepens the stretch, enhancing the mobility and flexibility of the shoulder joints.

5. Hold this position for several breaths, focusing on the stretch and release of tension in the upper body.

6. Slowly unwind your arms and repeat the exercise on the opposite side.

Targeted Areas:
Hips, thighs, and lower back.

SEATED LEG SWINGS

Benefits:

It enhances hip mobility and leg flexibility while improving circulation.

Safety Precautions:

• Swing your leg gently to avoid strain.

• Ensure the chair is stable.

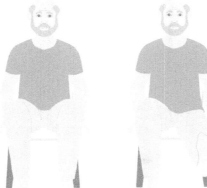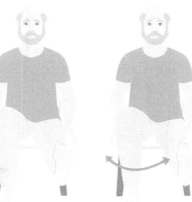

Steps:

1. Sit at the edge of a stable chair with your feet planted firmly on the floor. This starting position ensures a solid base and prepares your body for movement.

2. Grasp the sides of the chair with both hands for stability. This support is crucial for maintaining balance during the exercise.

3. Extend one leg forward, keeping it as straight as comfortable. This extension prepares your leg for the swinging motion.

4. Gently swing the extended leg from side to side, allowing it to cross in front of your stationary leg. This movement should be controlled and within a comfortable range to avoid strain.

5. Continue the swinging motion for 10-15 repetitions, focusing on smooth, fluid movements to maximize the stretch and mobility benefits.

6. After completing the swings with one leg, pause for a moment to reset, then switch to the other leg, repeating the swinging motion for 10-15 repetitions.

SEATED SPHINX POSE

Targeted Areas:
Spine, chest, and shoulders.

Benefits:

Designed for seniors to strengthen the spine, open the chest and shoulders, and potentially alleviate lower back pain. It supports improved posture and respiratory function.

Safety Precautions:

• Keep your movements gentle and avoid straining your lower back.

• If you have severe back issues, consult a healthcare professional first.

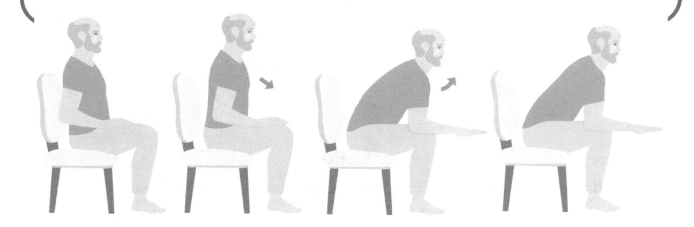

Steps:

1. Position yourself at the front edge of a chair, ensuring your feet are planted firmly on the ground, shoulder-width apart.

2. Initiate the movement by bending forward from your hips, keeping your spine straight to maintain its natural curvature.

3. Slide your hands down your thighs while gently lowering your elbows to rest them on your thighs, transitioning smoothly into the pose.

4. Adjust your position so your elbows are directly beneath your shoulders, forming a 90-degree angle with your arms. This alignment replicates the traditional Sphinx Pose while seated, focusing on spinal integrity and shoulder openness.

5. Slightly lift your chest, creating a gentle arch in your back. This movement emphasizes spinal extension and chest opening, enhancing the stretch.

6. Extend your neck forward, keeping it in line with your spine, to ensure a comprehensive stretch without straining.

7. Hold this position for 5 breaths, focusing on deep, steady inhalations and exhalations to support relaxation and effectiveness of the pose.

8. To conclude, gently raise your torso back to the starting position. Aim for up to 3 repetitions, each time focusing on maintaining smooth movements and proper alignment.

SEATED UPWARD ARM STRETCH

Targeted Areas:
Arms, shoulders, and side torso.

Benefits:

Designed to stretch the arms and sides, enhance posture, and alleviate mild back discomfort.

Safety Precautions:

• Stretch within your comfortable range.

• Avoid if you have severe shoulder pain.

OPTIONAL

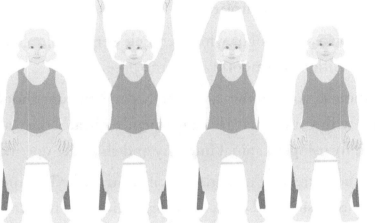

Steps:

1. Begin by sitting upright on a stable chair, feet grounded on the floor. This posture forms the foundation for a safe and effective stretch.

2. As you inhale, extend both arms overhead, ensuring your shoulders remain down and away from your ears to maintain relaxation in the neck.

3. For an added stretch, interlace your fingers and gently turn your palms upward, towards the ceiling. This intensifies the stretch along arms and sides of the torso.

4. Reach upwards as you keep your spine elongated, imagining each vertebra stretching away from the next. This action not only stretches the arms and sides but also encourages a tall, healthy posture.

5. Hold this uplifted position for a few deep breaths, allowing the stretch to deepen naturally with each exhale.

6. Gently lower your arms back to your sides as you exhale, feeling the release throughout your shoulders and arms.

Targeted Areas:
Shoulders, upper back, chest, and core muscles.

Benefits:

To enhance hip mobility and leg flexibility while improving circulation.

Safety Precautions:

• Move within a comfortable range to avoid shoulder discomfort.

• Keep your spine neutral to prevent undue strain on the back.

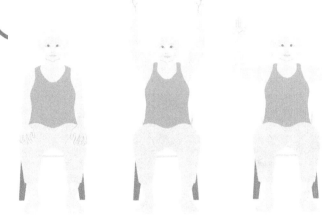

Steps:

1. Sit upright on a chair with feet flat on the ground, shoulder-width apart, providing a stable and supportive base.

2. Raise both arms towards the ceiling while engaging your core to stabilize your shoulders and ribcage.

3. Gently tuck your chin to maintain alignment of your head with your spine, avoiding forward head posture.

4. Exhale and bend your elbows, lowering your arms until they are parallel to the floor, with palms facing forward. Draw your shoulder blades together and gently lift your chest, creating the cactus arm shape.

5. Inhale and extend your arms back towards the ceiling, keeping your core engaged for stability and support.

6. Perform this bending and straightening motion 3-5 times, focusing on the movement's smoothness and the sensation of stretching and strengthening.

10 Day Chair Yoga Challenge

Now it's time to start the 10-Day Chair Yoga Challenge! The following pages will give you some instructions on how to get started, don't forget to get access to the video poses for extra guidance by scanning one of the QR codes that have been place throughout the book. Come join our Facebook community for motivation and extra support should you need it. Day 1 starts today, lets go!

Instructions:

Here are the steps to get started with your practice:

1. **Begin each day with a breathing exercise.** This will help to center your mind and prepare your body for the chair yoga session.

2. **Follow the sequence of poses as outlined for each day.**

3. **Take a short pause of 15 - 20 seconds between each exercise or pose.** Use this time to breathe normally and prepare for the next pose.

4. **Remember to go at your own pace.** It's important to listen to your body and not push beyond comfort. If you experience any discomfort, modify the pose or skip it as needed.

5. **Begin with the goal of practicing these chair yoga workouts daily.** I know that you're busy, but I've found that this consistent approach helps students to establish a routine and maximize the benefits of the program.

   » However, it's important to listen to your body and be mindful of your energy levels and physical comfort.

   » If you find that daily practice is too demanding, or if you experience any discomfort, it's perfectly fine to adjust your schedule.

   » This adjustment ensures that you still maintain regular practice while giving your body adequate time to rest and recover.

I'm here to support you on your journey to a healthier, happier life. If you have any questions, concerns, or would like a few words of encouragement, please don't hesitate to reach out (jcharrisonbooks@gmail.com).

Ending Each Session:

When you're finished with your yoga practice, take a few moments to meditate. This will help you to calm your mind and body and to integrate the benefits of your practice.

» Sit in a comfortable position in your chair. Close your eyes and take a few deep breaths. Focus on your breath, and let go of any thoughts or worries that come to mind.

» After a few minutes, you may want to try a simple meditation technique, such as focusing on a mantra or visualization. Or, you can simply sit quietly and enjoy the feeling of relaxation.

» When you're ready, open your eyes and slowly come back to the present moment. Take a few moments to appreciate the sense of relaxation and well-being that you've created.

On the next pages you will find a guide to follow. You can use the example poses provided or feel free to choose any pose you prefer from the list in this book.

Take a short pause of 15 seconds between each exercise or pose.

Three-Part Breath
(page 37).

Seated Neck Rolls
(page 47).

Chair Assisted Torso Twists
(page 53).

Seated Warrior II Arms
(page 56).

Seated Spinal Extension
(page 54).

Seated Side Stretch
(page 55).

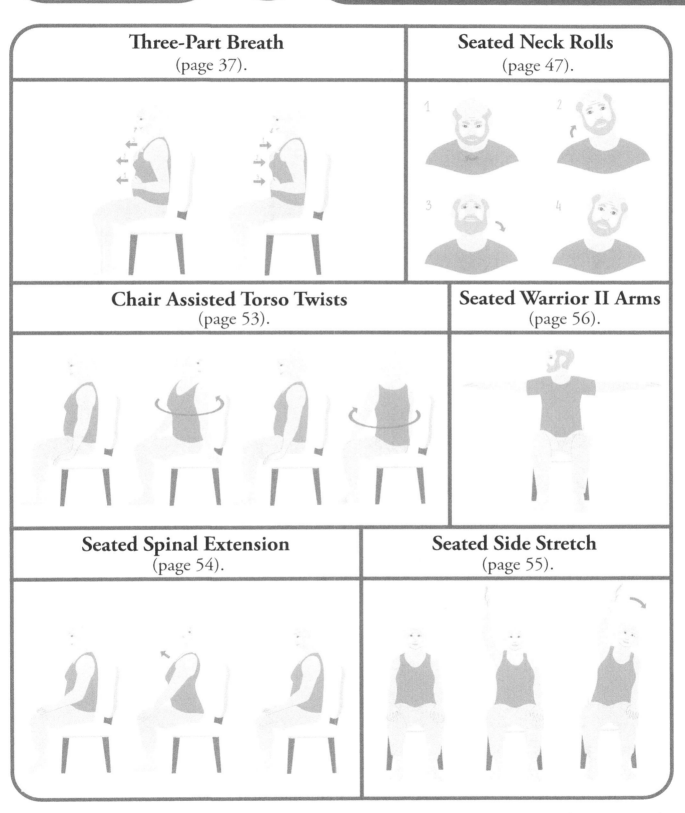

Take a short pause of 15 seconds between each exercise or pose.

Diaphragmatic breathing
(page 36).

Seated Arm Circles
(page 59).

Chair Cat-Cow Stretch
(page 60).

Seated Torso Circles
(page 63).

Chair Assisted Leg Lifts
(page 64).

Seated Forward Bend
(page 65).

Take a short pause of 15 seconds between each exercise or pose.

DAYS 6 - 8

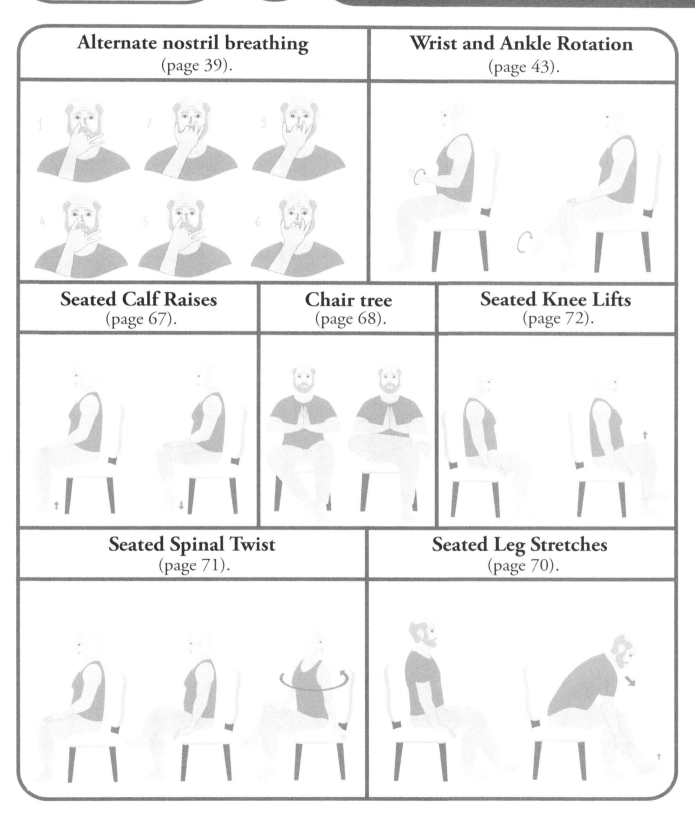

Alternate nostril breathing (page 39).

Wrist and Ankle Rotation (page 43).

Seated Calf Raises (page 67).

Chair tree (page 68).

Seated Knee Lifts (page 72).

Seated Spinal Twist (page 71).

Seated Leg Stretches (page 70).

Take a short pause of 15 seconds between each exercise or pose.

Ocean Breath
(page 38).

Shoulder Stretch
(page 45).

Chair Sun Salutation
(page 76).

Seated Knee Extensions
(page 78).

Take a short pause of 15 seconds between each exercise or pose.

Days 9 - 10 (Part II)

Chair Assisted Squats
(page 79).

Seated Jumping Jacks
(page 80).

Seated Sphinx Pose
(page 86).

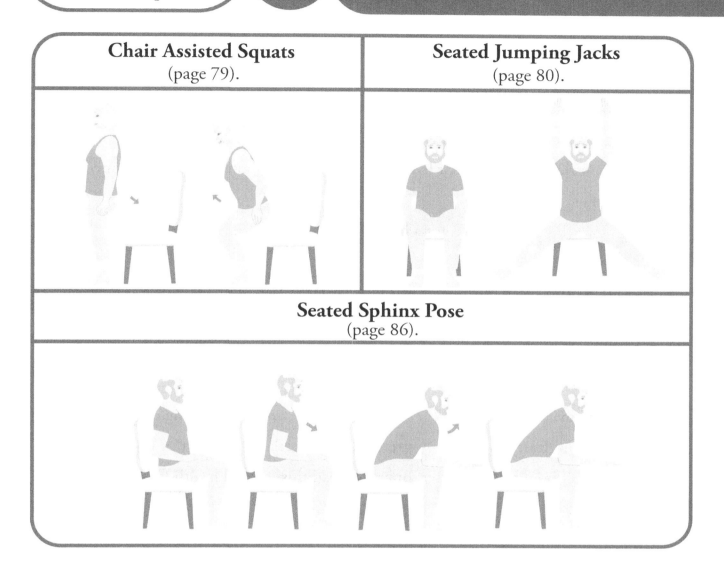

MAKE A DIFFERENCE WITH YOUR REVIEW

"Kindness, like a boomerang, always returns." – **Unknown**

Did you know that the kindest folks are often the happiest? It's true! When we do something nice for someone else, without thinking about what we'll get in return, we're sprinkling a little magic into their lives and ours. So, how about we sprinkle some of that magic together?

I've got a little favor to ask of you...

Imagine being able to help someone just like you, someone who once felt a bit unsure about starting something new, like chair yoga. Remember what it was like wanting to feel better, move easier, and enjoy life more, but not knowing where to start?

Our goal is to make *Chair Exercises For Seniors and Beginners* something everyone can enjoy and benefit from. Every move, every stretch, every breath we take in this book is aimed at making life a bit brighter and better. But, to spread this joy and health far and wide, we need your help.

Believe it or not, your opinion is super powerful. When someone is thinking about trying chair yoga, they look for what others have to say about it. So, here's my big ask on behalf of a friend you haven't met yet:

Would you share a few kind words about this book in a review?

It's a simple act that costs nothing and takes just a moment, but it could make a world of difference to someone looking for a sign to start their journey towards a more joyful and active life. Your review could help...

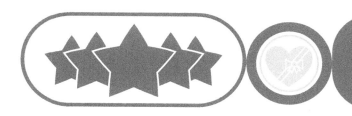

...another grandparent play freely with their grandkids.

...someone regain confidence in moving around their home.

...bring a smile to someone's face as they discover what they can achieve.

...inspire someone to start their journey to wellness.

To spread a little kindness and make a big impact, all you need to do is leave a review. It's easy: Simply go to https://geni.us/ChairExercises or scan the QR code below to share your thoughts or go to your orders on Amazon:

If the thought of helping someone out there warms your heart, then you're exactly the kind of person I wrote this book for. Welcome to our community of kindness warriors. You're one of us now.

I'm thrilled to be on this journey with you, helping you discover easier movements and brighter days through chair yoga. I can't wait for you to experience the joy and freedom waiting for you in the pages ahead.

Thank you from the bottom of my heart. Let's get back to our yoga adventure.

Your biggest cheerleader, *J.C. Harrison*

PS - Remember, sharing is caring! If you believe this book could help another soul dance through their day a little easier, why not share it with them? It's a simple way to spread joy and kindness, making you and the recipient feel great.

Movement is a medicine for creating change in a person's physical, emotional, and mental states.

– Carol Welch

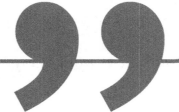

CHAPTER 5
MEDITATION AND CHAIR YOGA MADE EASY

Integrating meditation into your chair yoga routine offers a profound benefit, especially as we age. Meditation is a practice of focusing the mind on specific thoughts or experiences, a proven method for achieving a state of deep peace and relaxation. This mental discipline has roots stretching back thousands of years across various cultures, aimed at enhancing self-awareness, concentration, and spiritual growth. For seniors, the regular incorporation of meditation into daily life can be transformative, promoting mental clarity and a significant improvement in quality of life.

Research highlights meditation's ability to fortify neural pathways in the brain, crucial for memory retention and cognitive function, helping to mitigate age-related memory decline. Moreover, it boosts mood by increasing the production of serotonin and dopamine, the brain's natural feel-good chemicals. By consistently practicing meditation, you can also manage stress, lower levels of cortisol, the stress hormone, and maintain a serene and balanced mindset in everyday activities.

Meditation isn't just a practice, it's a transformation. As seniors, embracing meditation can be one of the most empowering decisions you make for your health and well-being. Keep this simple, remember this: meditation is about focusing the mind, and gently guiding your thoughts to create a haven of peace and clarity within you. This is not about becoming a Zen master overnight; it's about taking small, consistent steps towards a calmer, more centered you.

Unlocking a World of Benefits for Seniors

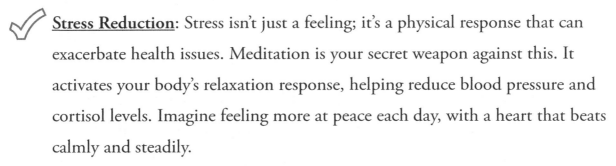

Stress Reduction: Stress isn't just a feeling; it's a physical response that can exacerbate health issues. Meditation is your secret weapon against this. It activates your body's relaxation response, helping reduce blood pressure and cortisol levels. Imagine feeling more at peace each day, with a heart that beats calmly and steadily.

Sharper Mind: Forgetfulness might seem like an inevitable part of aging, but meditation can help you sharpen your mind. It's like a workout for your brain, improving focus, attention, and memory. Picture your mind as a muscle that gets stronger and more resilient with each meditation session.

Emotional Resilience: Life's golden years should be just that – golden. Meditation helps in warding off feelings of loneliness or sadness, fostering a more positive and joyful outlook on life. It's about finding that inner strength and contentment, no matter what the day brings.

Pain Management: Many seniors struggle with chronic pain, but meditation can change your relationship with it. By focusing your mind, you can alter the way your body perceives pain, making it more manageable. It's about taking control, and not letting pain dictate your life.

✓ <u>**Restful Sleep**</u>: Those nights of tossing and turning? Meditation can help. By calming your mind, you pave the way for deeper, more restful sleep. Imagine waking up each morning feeling refreshed and rejuvenated.

✓ <u>**Improved Balance and Mobility**</u>: Meditation enhances body awareness, which in turn can improve balance and prevent falls. It's about being in tune with your body, moving through life with grace and confidence.

Incorporating meditation into your life is like planting a seed that grows into a tree of peace, resilience, and wellness. It's never too late to start. Each moment of mindfulness is a step towards a more vibrant, healthier you. Embrace this journey with an open heart and watch as your golden years become enriched with profound tranquility and joy.

Meditation: Your time, Your place

Choosing the right spot for meditation is key. Look for a quiet, peaceful area in your home where you can sit undisturbed. This could be a cozy corner or a spot with a pleasant view. The goal is to have a dedicated space that signals to your mind, "It's time to relax and focus." Consistency in your chosen spot helps in building a routine.

As for sitting, comfort is crucial. Use a sturdy chair that supports your back. Sit with your feet flat on the ground, hands resting gently in your lap. If needed, add cushions for extra support. The aim is to maintain a posture that's relaxed yet alert, ensuring you can focus without discomfort. Remember, in meditation, your comfort is the pathway to deeper focus and relaxation.

The perfect time to practice meditation is when it seamlessly fits into your routine, making it a sustainable and enjoyable habit. Here's the key: choose a time when you can be calm and undistracted, ensuring you get the most out of your practice.

Morning: Many find the early morning ideal, as the world is still quiet, allowing you to start your day with a clear, focused mind. It sets a positive tone for the day ahead.

Lunchtime or Breaks: A brief meditation session during lunch or on a break can be a great way to reset, especially if you're feeling stressed or overwhelmed.

Evening: If you need a way to unwind after a long day, evening meditation can be perfect. It helps you relax, let go of the day's stress, and improve sleep quality.

Before Bed: A short meditation before bed can aid in releasing the day's tensions, preparing your mind and body for a restful night's sleep.

Remember, the best time is when you can be consistent. Even just 5-10 minutes daily can make a significant impact. And don't forget, it's not just about fitting meditation into your schedule, but also embracing it as a moment of peace and self-care in your busy life. Let it be your personal retreat, a time when you prioritize your well-being and mental clarity.

To get you started with meditating I have included six different types of meditation practices that you can explore along with your chair yoga sessions.

MINDFULNESS BREATHING MEDITATION

Steps:

1. Choose a stable and comfortable place to sit (be it a chair, or bench). Ensure you're supported, not slouching or leaning. Place the soles of your feet flat on the ground.

2. Keep your back straight but relaxed, maintaining its natural curve. Let your head and shoulders rest naturally atop your spine.

3. Let your upper arms align with your body, then rest your hands on your legs. Find the middle ground—neither too far forward nor back.

4. Lower your chin slightly and allow your gaze to fall gently forward. You can close your eyes or keep them half-open, without focusing on anything specific.

5. Begin to Relax. Take a moment to relax into your position. Shift your attention to your breath or bodily sensations.

6. Notice the sensation of air moving in and out, choosing a point of focus (nose, belly, or chest). Mentally note "breathing in" and "breathing out."

7. When your mind wanders, gently bring your focus back to your breath. There's no need to stop thoughts, just return to your breathing.

8. If you need to move or scratch an itch, pause first. Choose intentionally when to adjust. Let thoughts and distractions come and go without engagement. Return to your breath each time without judgment.

9. When ready, gently lift your gaze (or open your eyes). Take in the sounds around you, feel your body, and acknowledge your thoughts and emotions. Pause, reflecting on how you wish to proceed with your day.

KEY TIP

Extend Mindfulness Beyond Meditation: Incorporate mindfulness into daily activities to deepen your awareness and presence in every moment.

Body Scan Meditation

Steps:

1. To get started lie down on your back on a comfortable surface. Ensure your body is in a straight line with arms resting at your sides, palms facing up. If lying down is uncomfortable, you can also do this seated in a chair.

2. Gently close your eyes to minimize distractions. This helps you focus more on internal sensations.

3. Breathe deeply and slowly a few times to initiate relaxation. Inhale through your nose, and exhale through your mouth, letting go of tension with each breath out.

4. **Start with Your Feet:** Focus your attention on your feet. Notice any sensations—warmth, coolness, pressure, tingling, or perhaps nothing at all. Breathe into your feet; as you exhale, imagine any tension melting away.

5. **Move to Your Legs:** Shift your focus up to your legs—calves, knees, and thighs. Observe any feelings or discomfort. With each exhale, release tension and let your legs relax completely.

6. **Notice Your Lower Back and Pelvis:** Bring awareness to your lower back and pelvis area. Breathe into these regions, relaxing muscles and releasing pressure as you exhale.

7. **Focus on Your Abdomen and Chest:** Pay attention to your abdomen and chest. Feel the rise and fall with each breath. Allow any tightness to dissolve with your out-breaths.

8. **Relax Your Shoulders and Neck:** Move your awareness to your shoulders and neck. These areas often hold a lot of stress. Breathe into them, and let the tension flow out as you breathe out.

9. **Pay Attention to Your Hands and Arms:** Notice any sensations in your hands and arms. Breathe in, directing your breath to these areas, and relax them fully as you breathe out.

BODY SCAN MEDITATION

Steps:

10. **Observe Your Face and Head:** Finally, focus on your face and head. Relax your jaw, cheeks, eyes, forehead, and the top of your head. Breathe in calmness and exhale any tension.

11. **Whole Body Awareness:** Expand your attention to include your whole body. Take a few deep breaths, feeling as if your entire body is breathing. With each exhale, release any remaining tension.

12. When you're ready, slowly bring movement back into your body by wiggling your fingers and toes. Gently open your eyes. Take a moment to notice how your body feels as a whole. Sit up slowly and transition back to your day.

KEY TIPS

<u>Be Gentle with Yourself:</u> If your mind wanders or if you lose focus, gently redirect your attention back to the body part you were focusing on.

<u>Don't Rush:</u> Move through each part of the body without hurry, allowing yourself to fully experience the sensations and relaxation.

WALKING MEDITATION

Steps:

1. Find a quiet, safe space where you can walk, either a path near your home or where you feel comfortable. This could be indoors or outdoors. The path doesn't need to be long, but it should allow you to walk without obstacles.

2. Stand at the start of your path. Close your eyes for a moment and set an intention for your practice. It could be anything that speaks to your current feelings, desires, or needs. It might be a word or a short phrase, such as "peace," "gratitude," "healing," or "being present." Your intention should resonate with you personally, reflecting something you wish to cultivate or acknowledge within yourself during the meditation. Take a few deep breaths to center yourself.

3. Gently open your eyes, maintaining a soft gaze. Be conscious of your surroundings but try to keep your focus inward.

4. Pay attention to your feet touching the ground. Feel the sensations in your soles as you lift one foot, move it forward, and place it down.

5. Begin to walk at a slower pace than usual. With each step, note the lifting, moving, and placing of each foot. This deliberate pace helps enhance awareness.

6. Sync your breathing with your steps, if possible. This might mean taking a step with each inhale and another with each exhale. Find a rhythm that feels natural to you.

7. Notice the sounds around you, the feel of the air on your skin, and anything you can see or smell. Acknowledge these sensations without getting attached to them.

8. If your mind wanders to other thoughts, gently bring your attention back to the act of walking and breathing. The goal is to stay present with each step and breath.

9. After completing your walk, stand still for a moment to reflect. Close your eyes and take a few deep breaths. Notice any sensations in your body or changes in your mind. Reflect on the sense of calm and presence you've cultivated.

10. **Open your eyes and gently transition back into your day, carrying the mindfulness and calmness with you.**

KEY TIPS

<u>Stay Relaxed</u>: Keep your body relaxed as you walk. Let your arms swing slightly if it feels natural.

<u>Use a Mantra</u>: If it helps, silently repeat a mantra or phrase with each step, such as "in" and "out" with your breaths, to help maintain focus.

<u>Adjust Your Pace</u>: The speed of your walking can vary based on what feels most conducive to mindfulness for you. Experiment with what helps you stay most present.

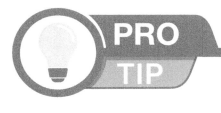

"Keep a Meditation Journal"

After meditating, spend a few minutes reflecting on your experience and jotting down any insights, challenges, or feelings. A journal can track your progress and deepen your understanding of your meditation journey.

LOVING-KINDNESS MEDITATION

Steps:

1. Choose a quiet and comfortable place to sit. You can sit in a chair with your feet flat on the ground. Ensure your back is straight but relaxed.

2. Gently close your eyes. Take a few deep breaths to relax. With each exhale, release any tension you're holding.

3. Start by focusing on a feeling of warmth and kindness towards yourself. You might visualize a gentle, warm light enveloping you or recall a moment when you felt loved and cared for.

4. Silently repeat phrases of loving-kindness towards yourself. Common phrases include:

May I be happy.

May I be healthy.

May I be safe.

May I live with ease.

5. Bring to mind someone you love deeply. Imagine directing feelings of warmth and kindness towards them. Silently recite the same phrases of loving-kindness towards this person.

6. Gradually extend your circle of kindness to include:

   » A good friend

   » A neutral person (someone you neither like nor dislike)

   » A difficult person (no need to start with the most difficult person)

Steps:

7. Finally, extend loving-kindness to all beings everywhere, without limitation.

8. For each new recipient, visualize them clearly and recite your phrases of loving-kindness. Try to genuinely wish them well and feel the warmth of your kindness extending to them.

9. After you have extended loving-kindness to all beings, sit quietly for a moment. Notice the feelings in your heart and body. Often, practitioners feel a sense of warmth, openness, or connectedness.

10. When you're ready, gently open your eyes. Take a moment to transition back into your day, carrying the feelings of loving-kindness with you.

KEY TIPS

Be Patient: Cultivating loving-kindness can take time, especially if you're dealing with feelings of self-criticism or resentment towards others.

Genuine Wishes: Aim for sincerity in your wishes. It's not just about repeating the phrases but truly wishing well for yourself and others.

Use Custom Phrases: Feel free to adapt the phrases to better suit you or to address specific wishes for yourself and others.

VISUALIZATION MEDITATION

Steps:

1. Find a spot where you can sit or lie down comfortably without interruptions. Ensure your environment is conducive to relaxation and focus.

2. Sit in a comfortable position with your back straight but relaxed, or lie down if you prefer. Use cushions or blankets as needed to support your posture.

3. Gently close your eyes. Take deep, slow breaths to relax your body. With each exhale, consciously release tension from your muscles.

4. Think about what you wish to achieve with your visualization. It could be a state of mind, like peace or happiness, or a specific goal you're working toward.

5. Begin to picture a scene in your mind that embodies your intention. This could be a place where you feel completely at peace, like a beach at sunset, a serene forest, or a cozy, safe space.

6. Make the visualization as vivid as possible by involving all your senses. See the colors and shapes, hear the sounds, smell the scents, feel the textures, and taste any flavors. For example, if you're visualizing a beach, feel the warmth of the sun on your skin, hear the waves crashing, smell the saltwater, and taste the fresh air.

7. As you deepen into the visualization, try to genuinely feel the emotions associated with your scene. Embrace the calm, joy, or satisfaction your visualization brings.

8. Spend several minutes immersed in your visualization, allowing the scene to evolve naturally. If your mind wanders, gently bring your focus back to your visualization.

9. When you feel ready to end your meditation, slowly bring your awareness back to the present. Take a few deep breaths and start to move your fingers and toes.

10. Gently open your eyes. Take a moment to transition back into your surroundings. Reflect on the experience and any feelings or insights that arose.

11. Try to maintain the sense of calm, focus, or well-being you cultivated during your visualization as you go about your day.

KEY TIPS

Flexibility: Your visualization can change and evolve; there's no need to stick rigidly to the first image that comes to mind. Let your imagination flow freely.

Practice Regularly: Like any form of meditation, the benefits of visualization grow with regular practice. Make it a part of your daily routine for the best results.

Use Guided Visualizations: If you find it challenging to maintain a visualization on your own, consider using guided visualization recordings that can help lead you through the process.

MANTRA MEDITATION

Steps:

1. Choose a peaceful place where you won't be disturbed. Sitting in a dedicated meditation space can enhance your practice, but any quiet spot will do.

2. Sit in a comfortable position with your back straight. Ensure your posture is alert yet relaxed.

3. Select a mantra that resonates with you. It can be a traditional Sanskrit phrase like **"Om Mani Padme Hum"** (the jewel is in the lotus) or a simple word or phrase in any language that holds personal significance, such as **"peace," "love,"** or **"I am calm."**

4. Gently close your eyes to minimize external distractions. This will help you focus inwardly and on the repetition of your mantra.

5. Take a few deep breaths to relax your body and mind. With each exhale, release any tension you're holding.

6. Silently repeat your mantra in your mind or whisper it softly. Your focus should be on the sound and vibration of the mantra as you recite it.

7. Continue to repeat your mantra at a pace that feels natural to you. There's no need to rush; allow the repetition to flow smoothly and steadily.

8. If you find your mind wandering to other thoughts, gently redirect your attention back to your mantra. The act of noticing distractions and returning to your mantra is part of the meditation process.

9. If you're concerned about time, set a timer for the duration you wish to meditate before you begin. This way, you can let go of the concern for time and fully immerse yourself in the practice.

10. When your meditation session is over, slowly cease the repetition of your mantra. Take a few deep breaths and gently bring your awareness back to your surroundings.

Steps:

11. Before opening your eyes, take a moment to notice the state of your mind and how you feel after the meditation. Acknowledge the peace and calm you've cultivated.

12. Open your eyes and take a moment to adjust. Move gently as you transition back to your daily activities, carrying the tranquility of your meditation with you.

KEY TIPS

Consistency Is Key: Regular practice enhances the benefits of Mantra Meditation. Aim to meditate at the same time each day to establish a routine.

Be Patient: It might take some time to notice the profound effects of your practice. Approach your meditation with patience and without expectation.

Personalize Your Practice: Feel free to adjust the length of your meditation sessions according to your comfort and schedule. Even a few minutes of dedicated practice can be beneficial.

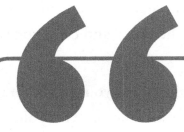

Self-care is how you take your power back.

– Lalah Delia

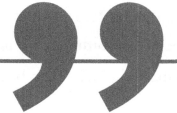

CHAPTER 6
THE ESSENTIAL GUIDE TO NUTRITION & CHAIR YOGA

Your Power Source in Senior Years

As we step into our senior years, it's time to turn a new page in our health story. Nutrition isn't just about eating; it's about fueling your life with the right energy. You might think it's too late to make changes, but I'm here to tell you it's not. Small shifts in your diet can lead to big wins in your health and vitality.

Nutrition's Impact: Why It's Crucial in Later Life

Remember, as we age, our bodies change. Our metabolism slows down, our digestive system may not be as efficient, and we might have different health concerns. But here's the good news: with the right nutrition, you can bolster your immune system, keep your bones strong, maintain your muscle mass, and feel more energetic. It's not just about adding years to your life, but life to your years!

THE BUILDING BLOCKS OF YOUR DIET

Let's talk about nutrition in a way that makes sense – no jargon, just straightforward facts. Your body is like a complex machine, and the food you eat is its fuel. Getting the right balance of nutrients is essential, but it doesn't have to be complicated. It's about getting back to basics and understanding the foundation of a healthy diet. These core principles are your allies in maintaining vitality and strength. Let's unravel these building blocks of nutrition, making each one simple and approachable. Whether it's the type of food you eat or the amount you consume, each element plays a crucial role in your overall health.

Let's simplify and look at what really matters:

Carbohydrates: Your Body's Primary Energy Source

Think of carbs as your body's main fuel. They break down into glucose (sugar in your blood), giving you the energy to keep moving.

> <u>Choose Wisely:</u> Opt for whole grains like brown rice or whole wheat, and don't forget fiber-rich fruits and veggies. These carbs are processed more slowly, providing a steady energy supply without the sugar spikes.

Whole Grains	Fiber-rich fruits
Brown rice, quinoa, whole wheat bread.	Apples, berries (such as blueberries or strawberries), oranges.

Proteins: The Building Blocks of Muscle and More

Protein isn't just for bodybuilders. It's crucial for repairing tissues, making hormones, and maintaining muscle mass – especially important as you age.

Quality Counts: Lean meats, fish, beans, and nuts are excellent choices. They provide essential amino acids without excess fat. Quality proteins are essential for maintaining and not losing muscle as you age.

Lean meats	Beans and legumes	Nuts and seeds
Chicken breast, turkey, lean cuts of beef.	Black beans, lentils, chickpeas.	Almonds, walnuts, pumpkin seeds.

Fats: Don't Fear Them, Understand Them

Fats have a bad reputation, but good fats are vital for brain health, energy, and absorbing vitamins.

Go for the Good Fats: Focus on unsaturated fats found in avocados, olive oil, and fatty fish like salmon. These can help reduce the risk of heart disease.

Avocados	Olive oil	Fatty fish
A great source of healthy monounsaturated fats.	Ideal for dressing salads or light cooking.	Salmon, mackerel, and sardines are high in omega-3 fatty acids.

Vitamins and Minerals: Your Secret Weapons

Think of them as your health's cheerleaders. Vitamin C boosts your immune system, Vitamin D is essential for bones, and B vitamins are key for energy.

Vitamins: From Vitamin A to Zinc, these little guys help keep your body functioning at its best. Focus on getting a colorful variety of fruits and vegetables to cover your bases.

Minerals: They're like the nuts and bolts keeping your body in top shape. Calcium and magnesium strengthen bones, iron is vital for healthy blood, and potassium helps control blood pressure.

Vitamin-rich fruits	Mineral-rich vegetables
Kiwi (rich in Vitamin C), bananas (potassium), cantaloupe (Vitamin A).	Spinach (iron and magnesium), broccoli (calcium and Vitamin K), sweet potatoes (Vitamin A and potassium).

Portion Control: Balance is Key

Eating the right amounts is just as important as eating the right foods. Listen to your body's hunger cues and remember, moderation is your friend.

A balanced plate: Half filled with vegetables, one-quarter with lean protein, and one-quarter with whole grains.

Snack portions: A small handful of nuts, a piece of fruit, or a cup of yogurt.

Fiber: more than just a dietary component

Fiber is a crucial player in your digestive health. Acting like a natural cleanser, fiber helps keep your digestive system running smoothly and efficiently. Often overlooked, fiber keeps your digestive system happy and can help manage blood sugar levels.

Incorporate fiber into your diet with choices like:

Whole grains, oats, fruits (like apples and pears), vegetables (like carrots and green beans), beans and legumes, such as lentils and chickpeas, are also excellent sources of fiber.

Hydration: The Elixir of Life

Water is crucial. It keeps everything running smoothly in your body. Not a fan of plain water? Try adding a slice of lemon or cucumber for a refreshing twist.

Water: The most straightforward and effective hydrator.

Herbal teas: Such as chamomile or peppermint, which are hydrating and can have additional health benefits.

Infused water: Adding cucumber, lemon, or berries to water for flavor.

Why Strengthening Bones and Muscles is Crucial

As we navigate our senior years, focusing on bone and muscle health isn't just a health recommendation; it's a necessity for active, independent living. Strong bones reduce the risk of fractures, and well-maintained muscles are essential for mobility, balance, and even simple daily tasks.

Bones: The Framework of Your Body: With age, bones can become more fragile due to a natural decline in bone density. A diet rich in calcium and vitamin D plays a critical role in maintaining bone strength and preventing osteoporosis.

Muscles: Your Source of Strength and Mobility: Muscle mass naturally decreases with age. However, consuming adequate protein and engaging in regular physical activity, like chair yoga, can help preserve and even build muscle strength.

Nutritional Keys for Bone and Muscle Health

Calcium	Vitamin D	Protein
It's the cornerstone for strong bones. Dairy products like milk and cheese, leafy greens like kale, and fortified foods are excellent sources.	Essential for calcium absorption, vitamin D can be obtained from the sun, but food sources like fatty fish, egg yolks, and fortified foods play a vital role, especially in colder climates or for those with limited sun exposure.	Crucial for muscle repair and growth. Options like lean meats, fish, beans, and nuts not only provide protein but are also packed with other nutrients beneficial for overall health.

Making It Pratical

Incorporating these nutrients into your daily meals can be both simple and delicious. Start your day with a Greek yogurt parfait, enjoy a spinach salad for lunch, and have grilled salmon for dinner. Snacks like a handful of almonds or cottage cheese can also be a tasty way to get your daily dose of bone and muscle-supporting nutrients.

Remember, what you eat directly impacts the strength and resilience of your bones and muscles. By choosing the right foods, you're not just eating; you're investing in your ability to live actively and independently.

Discover the Key to Longevity: Heart & Gut Health for Seniors

Maintaining a healthy heart and digestive system is more than just managing health; it's about enhancing the quality of life as you age. A strong heart ensures that your body gets the necessary nutrients and oxygen, while a well-functioning digestive system is key to absorbing these nutrients effectively. Together, they form the core of your well-being, influencing everything from energy levels to mood.

 Heart Health: As we age, our heart requires more attention. Eating heart-healthy foods can help manage blood pressure, reduce cholesterol levels, and lower the risk of heart disease.

 Digestive System: A robust digestive system aids in efficiently processing the food you eat, ensuring you reap the benefits of a nutritious diet. This is crucial for avoiding common age-related digestive issues.

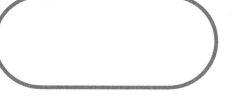

Nutritional Strategies for a Happy Heart and Gut

Oats and Whole Grains

Rich in soluble fiber, they help lower cholesterol levels and provide a steady source of energy.

Probiotic Foods

Yogurt, kefir, and fermented foods like sauerkraut help maintain a healthy gut flora, crucial for good digestion.

Berries and Antioxidant-Rich Foods

These help reduce inflammation and support heart health. Blueberries, strawberries, and raspberries are not only delicious but also packed with heart-healthy nutrients.

Leafy Greens and Fibrous Vegetables

Foods like spinach, kale, and broccoli are great for the heart and the digestive system, offering essential nutrients and fiber.

Why Energy and Immunity are Crucial in Senior Years

In our senior years, having consistent energy and a strong immune system isn't just a luxury; it's essential for enjoying life to its fullest. Sustained energy helps us stay active, engaged, and independent, while a robust immune system is our first line of defense against illnesses. The good news? Your diet plays a pivotal role in bolstering both.

Sustained Energy: As metabolism naturally slows with age, choosing the right foods can help maintain steady energy levels throughout the day.

Robust Immunity: With age, the immune system can weaken. A nutrient-rich diet supports its functioning, helping you stay healthier and recover faster from illnesses.

Diet Tips for Sustained Energy and Immunity

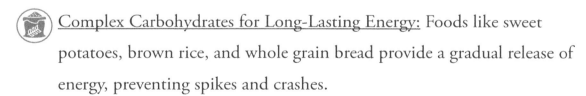 Complex Carbohydrates for Long-Lasting Energy: Foods like sweet potatoes, brown rice, and whole grain bread provide a gradual release of energy, preventing spikes and crashes.

Lean Proteins for Strength and Stamina: Incorporate chicken, turkey, fish, and plant-based proteins like beans and lentils. These help repair and build tissues, contributing to overall vitality.

<u>Antioxidant-Rich Fruits and Vegetables for Immune Support:</u> Citrus fruits, berries, bell peppers, and leafy greens are loaded with vitamins C and E, which bolster the immune system.

 <u>Healthy Fats for Energy and Cell Health:</u> Avocados, nuts, and olive oil provide essential fatty acids, supporting cell health and energy production.

Practical Ways to Boost Energy and Immunity

Regular, Balanced Meals	**Stay Hydrated**	**Snack Smart**
Eating at consistent times helps regulate your energy levels. Include a mix of carbohydrates, proteins, and fats in each meal.	Adequate hydration is key for energy and immune function. Aim for water, herbal teas, and hydrating foods like cucumbers and watermelon.	Choose snacks that combine protein and fiber, like apple slices with almond butter or yogurt with berries, for an energy and immune-boosting lift.

By focusing on these dietary strategies, you're equipping your body with the tools it needs to maintain high energy levels and a resilient immune system. This isn't just about food; it's about fueling your body for a joyful, active life in your senior years.

CONCLUSION

"Age is no barrier. It's a limitation you put on your mind."

– Jackie Joyner-Kersee

As we wrap up our chair yoga journey, it's time to reflect briefly on what we've accomplished together. This book isn't just information; it's your roadmap to a life filled with energy and positivity, no matter your age.

You now understand how to practice chair yoga comfortably and safely, equipped with techniques that can transform your daily experiences. Imagine navigating your day with ease, finding joy in routine tasks, and being an inspiration in every gathering. Chair yoga is more than exercise; it's a path to independence, health, and an optimistic view of life.

Crafted with love and intention, this book aimed to light a spark within you—to show that chair yoga is a golden key accessible to all, customizable to your unique rhythm, and immensely rewarding. With every pose you master, you'll feel yourself growing stronger, your body becoming more supple, and your balance steadier. Each small victory on the mat mirrors a giant leap toward a life that's richer and more vibrant.

Chair yoga is not just a routine; it's a testament to your strength and ability to adapt. Begin with enthusiasm, leverage the tools you've learned, and believe in gradual progress. This journey is about patience, celebrating each achievement, and staying committed. Keep refining your practice as you advance, making it a cornerstone of your health.

Let this book be more than a guide; let it be the dawn of a commitment to a practice that enriches every corner of your existence. Step into the embrace of chair yoga with an open heart and let it infuse your life with its transformative energy. Here's to you—stepping boldly into a future filled with health, happiness, and the joy of living life to the fullest, one breath, one pose at a time.

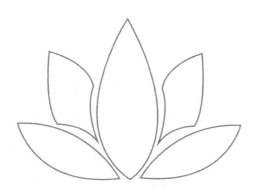

Now that you've embarked on this incredible journey with me, discovering the ease and joy of chair exercises, you're equipped with all the tools you need to embrace a life full of movement, flexibility, and peace. It's your turn to pass the torch and illuminate the path for others seeking the same serenity and vitality you've found.

By sharing your genuine thoughts about "Chair Exercises for Seniors & Beginners" on Amazon, you're not just leaving a review; you're guiding other seniors towards a gateway of transformation. Your words have the power to light the way for someone else in search of a brighter, more active, and joyful chapter in their life.

We're all part of a beautiful cycle of learning and teaching, giving and receiving. Your contribution by leaving a review keeps this cycle in motion, ensuring that the wisdom and benefits of chair yoga continue to enrich lives far and wide.

Thank you deeply for your support. The legacy of chair exercises thrives and expands with each story shared and each life touched – and you're playing a pivotal role in this beautiful journey.

Go to https://geni.us/ChairExercises or scan to leave your review on Amazon.

Your insights and experiences are invaluable, not just to us, but to the countless others on the cusp of discovering their own path to wellness through chair yoga. Together, we're not just practicing yoga; we're fostering a community of health, happiness, and shared knowledge. Thank you for being an essential part of this community and for helping to keep the spirit of chair yoga alive and flourishing!

Bao, W., Sun, Y., Zhang, T., Zou, L., Wu, X., Wang, D., & Chen, Z. (2020). Exercise Programs for Muscle Mass, Muscle Strength and Physical Performance in Older Adults with Sarcopenia: A Systematic Review and Meta-Analysis. Aging and Disease, 11, 863 - 873. https://doi.org/10.14336/ad.2019.1012.

Bonura, K., & Tenenbaum, G. (2014). Effects of yoga on psychological health in older adults. Journal of physical activity & health, 11 7, 1334-41. https://doi.org/10.1123/jpah.2012-0365.

Fishman, L. (2021). Yoga and Bone Health. Orthopaedic Nursing, 40, 169 - 179. https://doi.org/10.1097/NOR.0000000000000757.

Ghahramani, A. (2014). The effect of the relaxation training on the general health and selected physical fitness factors affecting seniors balance. Asian journal of multidisciplinary studies, 3.

Law, S., Leung, A., & Xu, C. (2021). Is Yoga possible for elderly care? Geriatric Care. https://doi.org/10.4081/GC.2021.9815.

Marciniak, R., Sheardová, K., Čermaková, P., Hudeček, D., Šumec, R., & Hort, J. (2014). Effect of Meditation on Cognitive Functions in Context of Aging and Neurodegenerative Diseases. Frontiers in Behavioral Neuroscience, 8. https://doi.org/10.3389/fnbeh.2014.00017.

McArthur, C., Laprade, J., & Giangregorio, L. (2016). Suggestions for Adapting Yoga to the Needs of Older Adults with Osteoporosis.. Journal of alternative and complementary medicine, 22 3, 223-6. https://doi.org/10.1089/acm.2014.0397.

McCaffrey, R., Park, J., Newman, D., & Hagen, D. (2014). The effect of chair yoga in older adults with moderate and severe Alzheimer's disease. Research in gerontological nursing, 7 4, 171-7. https://doi.org/10.3928/19404921-20140218-01.

Park, J., & McCaffrey, R. (2012). Chair yoga: benefits for community-dwelling older adults with osteoarthritis. Journal of gerontological nursing, 38 5, 12-22; quiz 24-5. https://doi.org/10.3928/00989134-20120410-01.

Park, J., Newman, D., McCaffrey, R., Garrido, J., Riccio, M., & Liehr, P. (2016). The Effect of Chair Yoga on Biopsychosocial Changes in English- and Spanish-Speaking Community-Dwelling Older Adults with Lower-Extremity Osteoarthritis. Journal of Gerontological Social Work, 59, 604 - 626. https://doi.org/10.1080/01634372.2016.1239234.

Park, J., Tolea, M., Rosenfeld, A., Arcay, V., Karson, J., Lopes, Y., Small, K., & Galvin, J. (2018). FEASIBILITY AND EFFECTS OF CHAIR YOGA TO MANAGE DEMENTIA SYMPTOMS IN OLDER ADULTS. Innovation in Aging. https://doi.org/10.1093/GERONI/IGY023.1142.

REFERENCES

Yao, C., & Tseng, C. (2019). Effectiveness of Chair Yoga for Improving the Functional Fitness and Well-being of Female Community-Dwelling Older Adults With Low Physical Activities. Topics in Geriatric Rehabilitation, 35, 248 - 254. https://doi.org/10.1097/TGR.0000000000000242.

You, S., Hong, S., & Moon, K. (2013). Effects of Hatha Yoga Practice on the Elderly Having Chronic Back Pain Because of Computer Usage. The Journal of the Korea institute of electronic communication sciences, 8, 1121-1128. https://doi.org/10.13067/JKIECS.2013.8.7.1121.

Made in the USA
Monee, IL
13 April 2025